W9-BNQ-750

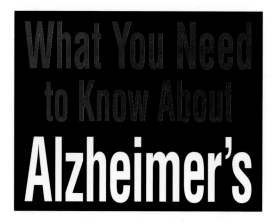

What You Need to Know About Alzheimer's

John Medina, Ph.D.

Foreword by John L. Schwartz, M.D.
Editor in Chief, *Psychiatric Times*

CME, INC.

NEW HARBINGER PUBLICATIONS

Publisher's Note
This publication is designed to provide accurate and authoritative information in regard to the subject matter covered. It is sold with the understanding that the publisher is not engaged in rendering psychological, medical, financial, legal or other professional services. If expert assistance or counseling is needed, the services of a competent professional should be sought.

Distributed in the U.S.A. by Publishers Group West; in Canada by Raincoast Books; in Great Britain by Airlift Book Company, Ltd.; in South Africa by Real Books, Ltd.; in Australia by Boobook; and in New Zealand by Tandem Press.

Published by CME, Inc. and New Harbinger Publications, Inc.

Cover design by Rick Tirabasso.
Text design by John Medina, Ph.D.

Library of Congress Catalog Card Number: 98-67410
ISBN 1-57224-127-6 Paperback

Printed in Hong Kong.

New Harbinger Publication's Website address: www.newharbinger.com
CME, Inc.'s Website addresses: www.mhsource.com and www.medicineandbehavior.com

First Printing

Dedicated to Cynthia and Kyle

Judy looked at me wild-eyed.

*"Do you know where my husband is?" she cried.
At first I just laughed, but as she turned more
anxious, grabbing my hand and shaking, I saw she
was serious. That's when I became speechless. The
reason for my reaction is that I am her husband.*

— Bill P., whose wife suffers from
Alzheimer's disease.

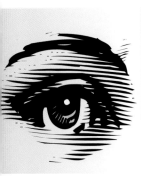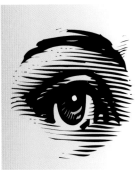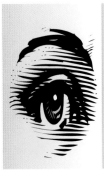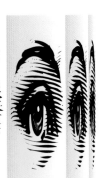

contents

1   **Introduction**

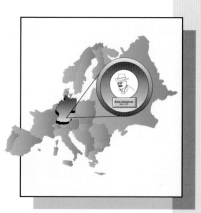

7   **PART ONE:**
Defining Alzheimer's
disease

9   **Chapter One**
The world of Alzheimer's disease

21   **Chapter Two**
What Alzheimer's looks like

41   **PART TWO:**
Discovering why
Alzheimer's destroys the brain

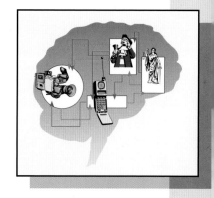

45   **Chapter Three**
Memory and the brain

57   **Chapter Four**
Nerve cells and the genetic code

81   **Chapter Five**
Why Alzheimer's destroys the brain

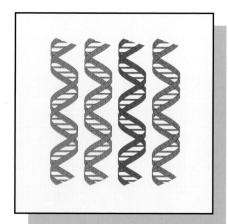

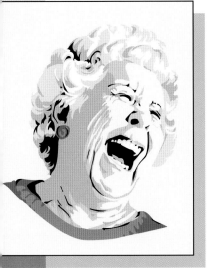

PART THREE:
Caring for the Alzheimer's patient: Practical suggestions

Chapter Six   **109**
Caring for the Alzheimer's patient

Chapter Seven   **119**
Living with Alzheimer's: practical suggestions

Appendix A   **148**
Other causes of Alzheimer's?

Appendix B   **150**
A cure for Alzheimer's disease?

Appendix C   **152**
Medical treatment of difficult behaviors

Appendix D   **154**
Alzheimer's by the numbers

Appendix E   **156**
What we are learning from nuns

Appendix F   **158**
Where to turn for help

Appendix G   **160**
Selected references

Index   **165**

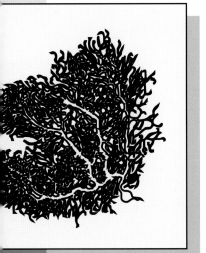

FOREWORD

Alzheimer's disease is relentlessly destroying the brains and lives of our nation's older adults, robbing them of memory and the ability to reason as well as affecting their emotions and behavior. The longer we live, the greater the risk: one out of every two Americans aged 85 and older and one out of every 10 aged 65 and older are afflicted with the disease. By the year 2050, an estimated 14 million Americans will be in its grip. Allen Roses, M.D., a researcher in the genetics of this disease, once noted that "We would all be at risk for Alzheimer's disease if we were to live to age 130 years."

John Medina, Ph.D., a research molecular biologist and professor at the University of Washington School of Medicine, provides a clear, comprehensive and compassionate view of this progressive and disabling disease. A one-time commercial artist, Medina uses the power of drawings and color to describe how the brain works, what Alzheimer's disease, with its plaques and tangles, looks like, and how it destroys brain cells. The ten major warning signs of the disease and research directions are also explored by Medina.

Recognizing that for each victim of Alzheimer's disease there is also a caregiver—usually a spouse or child—who must not only watch the decline but cope with their loved one's loss of memory, concentration, speech, ability to dress, bathe, walk, sit up or even smile, Medina provides practical suggestions. He discusses how to deal with difficult behavior, cope with specific kinds of memory loss, secure living quarters, handle grooming and other personal activities, make life more enjoyable for the person with Alzheimer's and plan for long-term care and medical crises. The family-friendly approach of the book is also enhanced by Beth's poignant journal entries of her "life with daddy," as he progresses through the stages of Alzheimer's disease.

Whether you, someone you love, or a friend is suffering from Alzheimer's disease, Medina suggests there is reason for hope. While there is no all-encompassing cure for Alzheimer's disease, several recent breakthroughs (vitamin E, estrogen, anti-inflammatory therapy, gene therapy, and existing medications such as tacrine and donepezil) hint that effective treatments may one day be available to everyone.

This is an important and fascinating book. I thank Dr. Medina for bringing this vital information to all of us.

—John L. Schwartz, M.D.
Editor in Chief
Psychiatric Times

Art, like morality, consists of drawing the line somewhere.

—G.K. Chesterton

I am a research molecular biologist and a teaching professor on the faculty of the University of Washington School of Medicine. Before I was an academic scientist, however, I was a professional graphic artist. For some people, to have those two professions resident in one person seems like a contradiction in terms. Science, a mind-numbingly tedious career punctuated by the occasional spine-tingling discovery, appears very different from any part of the rest of the world. Especially the creative arts.

This conundrum hints at something that is disturbing to many of us in our labs and classrooms. A gap of misunderstanding exists—and is widening—between scientists and the rest of society. We researchers speak our arcane language and the lay public politely listens, realizes the unintelligibility, shrugs its shoulders, and goes to the grocery store. There they purchase a newsmagazine like *Time* or *Newsweek* to provide articles that explain and clarify our discoveries—ones about which we researchers appear only to mumble.

This book is an attempt to close that growing and completely unnecessary gap. As a commercial artist, I long ago realized the power of pictures and color to convey clearly even the most convoluted and obscure ideas. This book attempts to use that power, with the full knowledge that nothing can seem more convoluted or obscure than research science. The pages are deliberately graphics-driven, and laid out in a style reminiscent not of a trade book, but of a newsmagazine. Studies in biology are not essential to understand the concepts. By the time the last page is reached, the reader will take away some of the most recent scientific thinking about the very crucial subject of Alzheimer's disease.

Speaking as both a scientist and a former graphic artist, I quite agree with G.K. Chesterton. And I hope that this book can fashion from that line something that also functions as a bridge.

—John Medina

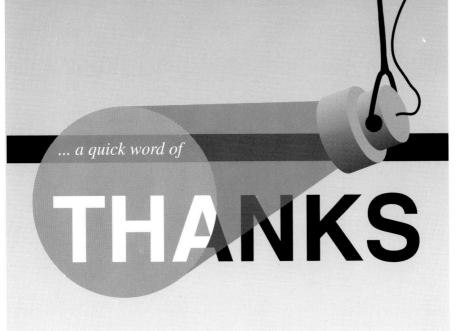

... *a quick word of*

THANKS

SPOTLIGHTING SOME VERY HELPFUL PEOPLE

With gratitude I acknowledge the editorial assistance, wisdom, gentle cajoling, and warmth of my editor, Ronald Pies, M.D. I would also like to express my gratitude to John L. Schwartz, M.D., and David DeNinno for their vision for this project and their long-standing friendship. My thanks go to Sandy Somers, Rick Tirabasso and Ken Hammond, without whom this book would not have been possible.

As ever, I would like to acknowledge the love and unflagging support of my wife, Kari, whose friendship and patience, after all these years, is still as fresh and immediate as the day we met. You, my dear, are amazing.

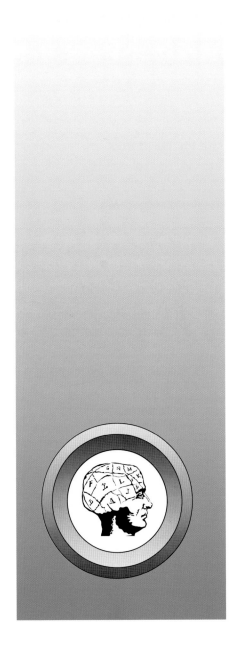

INTRODUCTION

Portraits of Alzheimer's disease

Alzheimer's disease is a degenerative disorder of the brain. It affects two groups of people: those with the disease and the loved ones who care for them.

THE PICTURE BOX

We used to joke about Carol's inability to remember details. As we got older, her memory got worse, but since I had trouble recalling things too, neither of us greatly worried. One day Carol and I went to the mall to buy a dress. As we approached the store, she suddenly forgot where we were going, or even where we were. This disorientation agitated her greatly and it took several minutes to calm her down. Eventually Carol remembered the dress; we found the store, bought the item and went home.

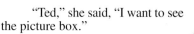

Though that situation bothered me, I felt no real alarm until a week later. Carol came into my study, a worried look on her face. The conversation that followed was so startling that I jotted it down.

"Ted," she said, "I want to see the picture box."

"Do you mean the television, dear? The computer?"

"No, it makes pictures."

"Carol, can you tell me what it looks like?"

"It looks like a box of nails."

At that point my wheels were turning. Pictures? A box shape? Did Carol mean our Polaroid?

"Do you mean the camera, Carol?"

"That's it. I want the camera."

At that point I knew something was terribly wrong. Over dinner I suggested we call a doctor, but Carol was resistant. Later that evening I discussed the situation with our daughter, who had also noticed unusual behavior. She came over the next day and together we talked to Carol, who reluctantly agreed to see a specialist. The next month was the hardest I have experienced in our 39 years of marriage. After a seemingly endless series of tests, with no one committing to a definite diagnosis, we got a phone call from our doctor. He said that Carol was probably in the early stages of Alzheimer's disease, and I did not hear the rest of what he said because I dropped the phone and began to cry.

A BELL NAMED NANCY

Susan lovingly handled her father's early bouts with Alzheimer's. Though he had problems recalling simple things, like swallowing after he had chewed a mouthfull of food, life had more or less a predictable routine. Sometimes her father would burst out crying for no apparent reason. At those times, Susan would go to the piano and start playing songs from his favorite Broadway musicals. Invariably he would stop crying, and in a fine deep bass voice begin singing with Susan. Sometimes they played and sang for hours.

Lately, however, Susan's father appears to have gotten worse. Several weeks ago he began walking around the house like he was restlessly searching for something. Room to room he would wander, sometimes silent as a ghost, other times noisy, disturbing books, papers, even pulling the sheets from made-up beds. He began crying out for his wife, Nancy, who had died in Susan's childhood. He would search every square inch of his home, calling Nancy's name.

One day while Susan was upstairs, her father wandered outside. Through the window, she saw him starting to cross the street. Susan rushed outside, grabbed him by the shoulders, pulled him back inside. He explained that he was off to visit a friend in New England. As his wandering grew worse, a friend suggested that Susan hang a bell over the outside doors. She could then tell when he exited, even if she wasn't close by. Not wanting to keep her father a prisoner, but still wanting him safe, Susan agreed. She named the little bell Nancy.

A BROKEN ROSE

My best friend, Rachel, finally put her mother, Connie, in a nursing home. And I have never felt so bad for anyone in my life.

For years she had put up with the familiar Alzheimer's ravages—loss of memory, disorientation, wanderings, even diapers. Once Rachel found her mom eating mashed potatoes and peas with her fingers. Though she considered herself shock-proof, Rachel was stunned to realize that Connie had forgotten how to use a knife and fork. She tried teaching her mother, and for a few days Connie successfully imitated her. But she forgot frequently, and Rachel eventually just fixed foods Connie could eat with her hands.

The hardest things for Rachel were not the deteriorating bodily functions, bad as they could be, but her mother's increasingly dangerous mood swings. One evening Connie threw her food at a wall and screamed at the top of her lungs, "You're trying to poison me!" No amount of explanation could convince Connie otherwise. Though her mom eventually settled down, Rachel neared the breaking point. The next night Connie did the same thing, this time throwing a dish.

Rachel called me that night and just sobbed. She was wracked with guilt because caring for her mother was beginning to be more than she could bear. For the millionth time I suggested she look for some kind of assisted living situation. This time Rachel put up no argument. It took a great deal of time to find just the right place; there were huge waiting lists with which to contend. But eventually Connie found a home. I sent Rachel a card with a rose that said, "Troubles are like a flower, God never lets one bloom on a stem too weak to handle it." Rachel broke the rose, putting the stem in the trash. Later she called to say thank you and then to apologize.

Our approach to describing Alzheimer's disease

The book you have in your hands seeks to explain the behaviors of the three people described on the previous page. Each person is in a different stage of Alzheimer's disease (also called AD), with characteristic deterioration of nerve cells within their brains. This book discusses the symptoms, causes and treatments of the illness, which afflicts more than 4 million Americans today. The organization of the text, divided into three sections, is described below.

DEFINING ALZHEIMER'S DISEASE

WHAT?

We begin this section on a historical note, detailing how the ancients viewed memory disorders, describing how Alzheimer's was discovered in the twentieth century. We then attempt to define what exactly the disease is. As other disorders can mimic Alzheimer's, we will find this characterization no easy task (it can also be difficult to separate true Alzheimer's from the normal aging process, since the onset of the disease is often gradual and usually occurs in older populations). We then explain some of the warning signs that may point to the real thing, and describe what a doctor must do in order to arrive at the proper diagnosis. We end the section by detailing the progression of the disease as the years go by, explaining what to expect in terms of moods, behaviors and medical problems.

DISCOVERING WHY ALZHEIMER'S DESTROYS THE BRAIN

WHY?

This section describes why Alzheimer's inflicts its damage on human brains. We begin with a review of certain biological concepts: brain anatomy, memory mechanisms and how nerve cells and genes interact. This backdrop is used to explain what researchers find when they study the brains of Alzheimer's patients. We go deep into the nerve cells, peering into the dark, mysterious world of their genes and chromosomes. By relating this information to the outer behavior experienced by Alzheimer's patients,we attempt to illustrate the "whys" of disease progression. We also use this background to clarify current research directions, discovering that genes for several types of Alzheimer's exist. We also discuss the heritability of the disorder, explaining what genes and even environmental influences (if any) may predispose a person to acquire the disease.

PRACTICAL SUGGESTIONS FOR CAREGIVERS

HOW?

The final section addresses the more pragmatic issues of Alzheimer's disease: learning how to care for a person with the disorder. The section is divided into two parts. The first discusses general principles about caring for people with Alzheimer's, such as dealing with difficult behaviors and understanding the world in which an Alzheimer's patient lives. The second part focuses on the person directly, considering how to best interact with a loved one at various stages of the disease. Topics include how to manage memory and communication problems, physical and personal hygiene issues, mealtime management, exercise, structuring a day and dealing with death. Appendices at the end of the book have topics ranging from medical treatment for the disease to names and phone numbers of assistance-oriented national organizations.

Excerpts from a journal

In an effort to give as clear a view as possible, we spend considerable time in this book describing a seemingly detached disease process. It must be remembered, however, that the story of Alzheimer's is a very human one. We have thus included throughout the text excerpts from a fictionalized diary of a woman I will call Beth. The eldest daughter of a pediatrician, she watched her father slowly disintegrate because of Alzheimer's, and kept a journal detailing the experience. She has two younger siblings, Amy and Bill, who like Beth are grown and living away from home. Beth first became alarmed when her father gave her a phone call from his car. He had forgotten how to get home, even though he was downtown and in familiar territory. Here is her first entry, dated April 10, 1987.

I finally got Daddy to agree to visit Dr. Kramer. He only consented because of their long years of friendship. I called Kramer in advance and told him about the car incident, just in case Daddy was vague on the details. Amy was as ballistic as ever. I don't think she sees anything wrong, and she practically accused me of seeing spooks. Bill was still out of town. I feel really guilty, but Daddy's lack of memory scares me. Anyway, I'm glad I did it. I plan on taking him to the appointment myself, though I don't think he's happy about the idea. I know he senses something is wrong, and he has become withdrawn from practically everybody. I hope Kramer can sort this stuff out.

Just mentioning the appointment puts Daddy in a foul mood, and yesterday he had such a look on his face! He almost looked scared. Daddy has always been the strong one in the family and I have never seen him weak or afraid before. Amy and I were talking the other day and both of us can only recall seeing him cry once, when Mother died, and even then he closed the door to hide it from us. I think Amy is scared too, though she has a funny way of showing it. I fear the worst.

what

**defining
Alzheimer's
disease**

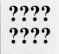

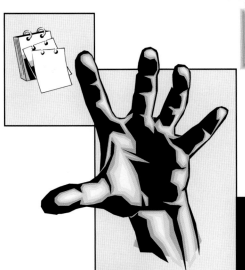

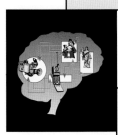

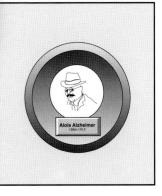

- *Alzheimer's throughout history*

- *Ten major warning signs of Alzheimer's disease*

- *The difficulty of diagnosis*

- *What happens when you visit the doctor*

- *The outward signs of Alzheimer's disease*

- *Behavior problems*

- *Mood problems*

- *Medical problems*

- *Death and Alzheimer's disease*

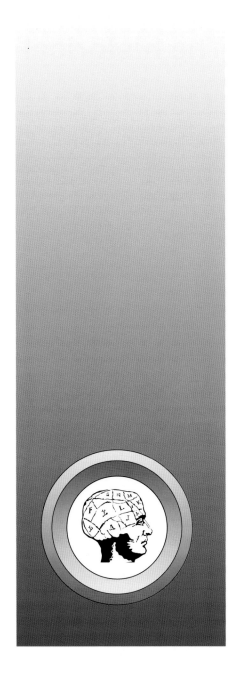

CHAPTER
ONE

*The world of
Alzheimer's disease*

The historical Alzheimer's

Though the idea of Alzheimer's disease is a fairly modern concept, there is evidence its symptoms were familiar in antiquity.

Many diseases that have acquired modern names were well-known before the twentieth century. Before we begin our discussion of modern-day Alzheimer's disease, it might be useful to answer a history question: Was Alzheimer's a disease familiar to people before its "discovery" in the twentieth century? The answer to this question is not easy to determine. The rigorous scientific standards required of medical investigators are really phenomena of the last hundred years or so. It has only been in the twentieth century that human life expectancy has increased sufficiently for researchers to examine meaningfully the diseases of old age. Despite these obstacles, scholars believe archeological evidence exists indicating that long-term age-related forgetfulness was known to the ancient world.

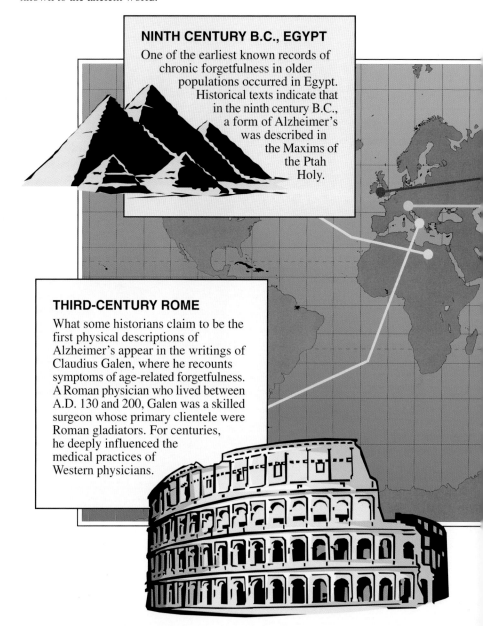

NINTH CENTURY B.C., EGYPT

One of the earliest known records of chronic forgetfulness in older populations occurred in Egypt. Historical texts indicate that in the ninth century B.C., a form of Alzheimer's was described in the Maxims of the Ptah Holy.

THIRD-CENTURY ROME

What some historians claim to be the first physical descriptions of Alzheimer's appear in the writings of Claudius Galen, where he recounts symptoms of age-related forgetfulness. A Roman physician who lived between A.D. 130 and 200, Galen was a skilled surgeon whose primary clientele were Roman gladiators. For centuries, he deeply influenced the medical practices of Western physicians.

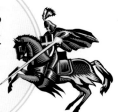

FOURTEENTH-CENTURY ENGLAND

A form of Alzheimer's also appears to have been known in the medieval era. A verbal exam that seems to screen for a kind of forgetfulness has even been uncovered. A series of questions given to Emma de Beston of Cambridge, England in 1383 was as follows (paraphrased):

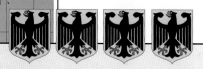

1) What town are you living in?
2) How many husbands do you have?
3) How many days are in a week?
4) How many shillings are in 40 pence?
5) Would you rather have 20 silver groats or 40 pence?

NINETEENTH-CENTURY GERMANY

It would be many centuries after Emma took her test that mental deterioration would be described in scientifically meaningful terms. The word *dementia* (meaning any psychological aberration associated with long-term brain disease) was first used by the famed German scientist Emil Kraepelin. He eventually described two major mental illnesses, which he called *manic depressive psychosis* and *dementia praecox*.

Kraeplin's influence on the field of psychiatry was enormous, and for two reasons. He was the first person to bring true scientific rigor to psychiatric illnesses. Before him, no one even knew if a physical disease were present in a mentally disturbed person. The second reason for his influence was his ability to surround himself with brilliant, inspiring colleagues. One of the researchers with whom he worked was to change the way we look at mental deterioration in older people. His name was Alois Alzheimer.

How Alzheimer's disease got its name

Though AD remains difficult to diagnose, it was not even considered a disease process until the early part of this century. For that, we can thank Alois Alzheimer.

Alois Alzheimer was a gifted German scientist who was born in the mid-nineteenth century. Though he will be forever linked to the disease that bears his name, Dr. Alzheimer actually did his landmark work in other areas of research. He was the first to link certain forms of senility, for example, with the accumulation of substances in the bloodstream. The sole reason his name became a household word for AD was because of a brief talk he gave to a small group of researchers in 1906. That presentation was published as an obscure note the next year. Below are some highlights of that presentation:

Dr. Alzheimer was examining a 51-year-old woman who was experiencing an unusual form of amnesia. He had been following her case for a number of years, and would later do an autopsy on her brain. Here is a quote from an English translation of the actual paper, describing her behavior:

When the doctor showed her some objects, she first gave the right name for each, but immediately afterwards she had already forgotten everything ... In her conversation, she often used confused phrases, single paraphrasic expressions (*milk-jug*, instead of cup). Sometimes she would stop talking completely. She evidently did not understand many questions (and) ... she did not remember the use of particular objects.

The woman died four years later, and when Dr. Alzheimer examined her brain, he found that many of her brain cells had totally disappeared. And then he made two startling discoveries. Here's the first one:

Inside an apparently normal-looking (nerve) cell, one or more single fibers could be observed that became prominent through their striking thickness. At a more advanced stage ... they accumulated, forming dense bundles.

He noticed that eventually the cells disappeared, and only the dense bundles, called *tangles*, remained. It was puzzling to see such bundles at all, but especially in someone so young. Dr. Alzheimer was a careful investigator, and he noticed something else besides the tangles. It became his second discovery:

Dispersed over the entire cortex, and in large numbers, (were) peculiar formations.

These peculiar formations, eventually called *plaques*, were different from the tangles. Like the tangles, the plaques had also not been found before in someone so young. There were thus two phenomena associated with this 51-year-old woman. Dr. Alzheimer did not know it at the time, but he was describing the brain of a person with a now-famous disease, one that would bear his name.

FURTHER STUDIES

Dr. Alzheimer eventually published the results of a second case in 1911, four years before he died. The twin observations of odd tangles and persistent plaques in senile patients became intriguing to more and more people. And also became more and more controversial. What was the nature of these tangles and plaques? Which came first, the behavior of Alzheimer's disease or the loss of nerve cells? Intriguingly, some of these questions remain a source of controversy (though as we'll see in a future chapter, some issues are becoming clearer). It is a testimony to the difficulty of this research that not much more was learned about Alzheimer's disease until relatively recently.

> **Why the nerve damage Dr. Alzheimer discovered occurs in human brains is still a mystery.**

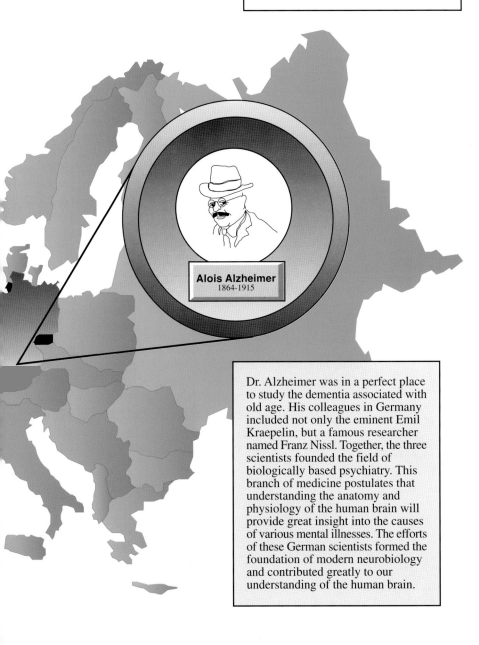

Alois Alzheimer
1864-1915

Dr. Alzheimer was in a perfect place to study the dementia associated with old age. His colleagues in Germany included not only the eminent Emil Kraepelin, but a famous researcher named Franz Nissl. Together, the three scientists founded the field of biologically based psychiatry. This branch of medicine postulates that understanding the anatomy and physiology of the human brain will provide great insight into the causes of various mental illnesses. The efforts of these German scientists formed the foundation of modern neurobiology and contributed greatly to our understanding of the human brain.

The ten major warning signs of Alzheimer's disease

There are a number of behaviors which may signal that a person might be in the beginning stages of Alzheimer's disease. Here's a list of warning signs:

A CHECKLIST

The research of Dr. Alzheimer initially described only a few of the many symptoms AD patients may experience. A great deal has been learned since his time about the early stages of the disease and accompanying behavior changes. Alterations in a person's thought life, actions, mood, and disposition can indicate the presence of AD. These days, professionals in the field have developed a list of warning signs that serve as a guide to determine if help is needed. Grouped into ten categories, they are described below (and will be explained in greater detail in the next chapter). Though these warning signs accurately describe the disorder, they are not necessarily predictors of AD. Such changes may be only the outward manifestations of normal aging, or may indicate disorders other than Alzheimer's (for example, depression can mimic Alzheimer's). Nonetheless, if some of these symptoms describe someone you know, the person may need to be professionally evaluated.

---

1. DIFFICULTY WITH FAMILIAR TASKS

It can be increasingly difficult for people with Alzheimer's disease to perform familiar duties. It is normal for people with busy schedules to go to a grocery store and forget to bring home, say, the Kleenex. People with AD may not only neglect the Kleenex, but may walk out of the store without paying for other purchases.

---

2. SLIPPING JOB PERFORMANCE

Going into a room and forgetting why you went, or losing a colleague's phone number only to remember it later can be a normal part of a business day. People with Alzheimer's begin to forget items or events much more often, and may not remember them at a later point. Eventually such memory lapses negatively affect job performance.

---

3. LANGUAGE DIFFICULTIES

People with Alzheimer's disease can begin to have problems with language. Unaffected people can have trouble remembering a person's name, or finding the right word in a social encounter. People with AD, however, may completely forget normal words in a sentence, or phrase words in such a fashion that their speech becomes incomprehensible.

---

4. CONFUSION OF PLACE AND TIME

Those with Alzheimer's disease can lose their sense of place and time. It is a normal part of living to occasionally lose track of time or to momentarily forget where you are. But individuals with AD can forget what year it is. They can become lost in their own homes, and not recognize loved ones they may have known for decades.

5. LACK OF JUDGMENT

Alzheimer's patients can exhibit increasingly poor judgment about activities of daily living. They might observe a loved one preparing a salad, and then attempt to help them by shredding newspaper on the kitchen table and placing it into the bowl. An individual with AD might put a dress on backwards, or walk down the interstate at two in the morning.

6. PROBLEMS IN ABSTRACT THINKING

An individual with Alzheimer's may have problems with abstract reasoning, such as doing simple mathematics. Many of us might find balancing our checkbooks or manipulating fractions in a recipe daunting tasks. Alzheimer's patients may not only have trouble with bank accounts, they may forget what addition is, or even what numbers are used for in normal society. Additionally, they may lose so-called executive functions, such as the ability to plan or strategize.

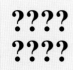

7. MISPLACING OBJECTS

A person with Alzheimer's may have difficulty putting objects away, or remembering where something is stored. Most people forget their car keys or misplace checkbooks from time to time. Someone with Alzheimer's, however, may put their wallet in the freezer or look for their glasses in the family aquarium, and appear to think this to be perfectly normal behavior.

8. MOOD FLUCTUATIONS

It is a familiar part of the human condition to feel melancholy or moody from time to time. An individual with Alzheimer's can exhibit extremely rapid emotional outbursts, however. These might start with sudden laughter followed by extreme anger and shouting and end with wracking sobs, all experienced with no apparent rhyme or reason.

9. CHANGES IN PERSONALITY

People with AD can undergo dramatic changes in personality and disposition. A person with AD who may have been cheerful and outspoken may turn confused, timid, and frightened. Some people with Alzheimer's disease become irreversibly suspicious of everyone they meet, including members of their families.

10. LACK OF INITIATIVE

Alzheimer's patients can exhibit passivity and lack of energy, even about important things. Anybody can tire of the daily stresses and strains of work and home. But people with AD may require constant prompting and encouragement to get involved in even the simplest tasks of daily living. They may forget to go to the bathroom; they may even chew their food but forget to swallow.

Alzheimer's disease is difficult for doctors to diagnose

The symptoms of Alzheimer's disease can mimic a number of other diseases. Here are some of the disorders with which AD can be confused.

ONCE IT WAS CALLED SENILITY

Though the ten warning signs listed may seem straightforward, Alzheimer's can be very hard for physicians to detect.There are several reasons for this. First, the symptoms of AD can look very similar to the symptoms of other disorders. Moreover, memory loss, a seemingly telltale sign of AD, is also a quite natural fact of old age. Physicians have even given this kind of memory loss a name: it is termed *age-associated memory impairment*. Such change is not indicative of disease, but simply of tenure on the planet.

There are, however, losses of intellectual skill that are not a normal part of the aging process. These can be severe enough to interfere with routine daily activities. A person may continuously forget to tie his shoes in the morning, for example, or may lose the skill altogether. Others may start looking for someone in their home who has either long since moved away or is dead. Adults who exhibit this abnormal behavior used to be called senile. These days, we simply call the syndrome *dementia*. As seen below and on the adjacent page, dementia can have many causes, with Alzheimer's being only one.

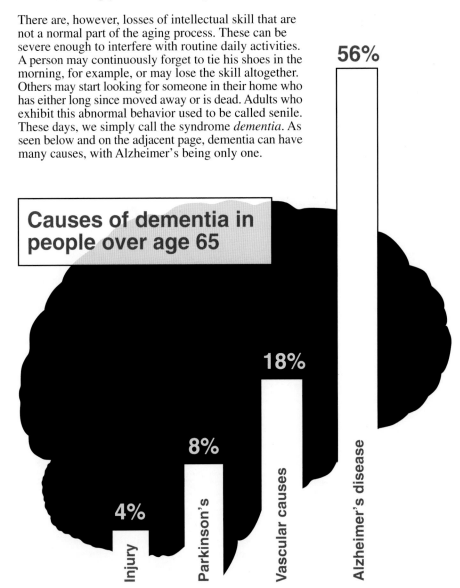

Causes of dementia in people over age 65

56% Alzheimer's disease

18% Vascular causes

8% Parkinson's

4% Injury

DISEASES THAT CAUSE DEMENTIA

Even though Alzheimer's disease is responsible for more dementia than all other causes combined, more than 60 other diseases are capable of causing AD-like dementias. That is why AD can be so hard to detect. It is also the reason why a physician must administer an exhausting battery of tests before making an Alzheimer's diagnosis. Below is a partial list of diseases the physician has to rule out, disorders which can cause dementias reminiscent of Alzheimer's disease.

MULTI-INFARCT DEMENTIA	Also called *vascular dementia*, this mental degeneration is caused by multiple strokes (physicians call strokes "infarcts") and is often associated with hypertension. Curiously, one-quarter of people who suffer from Alzheimer's disease also suffer from vascular dementia.
PICK'S DISEASE	This disease is a relatively rare brain deterioration, affecting a part of the brain known as the frontal lobe. It can closely mimic the symptoms of Alzheimer's. Like AD, it can be very difficult to diagnose: absolute certainty of the presence of Pick's disease is usually not obtained until an autopsy is performed.
CREUTZFELD-JAKOB DISEASE	A fatal brain disease, Creutzfeld-Jakob disease is caused by an infectious agent, probably a virus. Lack of coordination, failing memory, and mood changes are observed early in the disease's course. Death usually ensues within a year of the initial diagnosis
PARKINSON'S DISEASE	People with Parkinson's have low levels of an important brain chemical called dopamine. Symptoms include tremors and a general slowing of motor activity; only in the late stages of the disease is dementia observed. Some Parkinson's patients develop Alzheimer's disease, just as some AD patients develop Parkinson's.
MAJOR DEPRESSION	Clinical depression is characterized by lethargy, deep sadness, difficulty in concentrating, suicidal thoughts, and other symptoms. A percentage of severely depressed patients experience dementia. Alone among the various dementias, this form can be completely reversed with proper treatment.
ACQUIRED IMMUNE DEFICIENCY SYNDROME	The human immunodeficiency virus (HIV) can attack nerve cells in the brain. Intellectual deterioration occurs when enough nerve cells are destroyed. AIDS-associated dementia is usually seen in the later stages of the disease.

Other diseases that cause dementia include brain tumors, liver and kidney failure, chronic alcoholism, blood clots in the brain, late multiple sclerosis, posttraumatic brain injury, even late-stage syphilis. With the variety of diseases capable of creating dementias, it is small wonder that determining the presence of Alzheimer's can take a long time.

What happens on the visit to the specialist

Because of the difficulty detecting AD, a physician usually has to order a large battery of tests. These are designed to rule out other explanations for the observed dementia.

NEVER-ENDING TESTS

Determining the presence of AD can be a frustrating experience. This is because no *one* test can determine whether Alzheimer's actually exists. In fact, the only way to absolutely prove AD is to examine the actual brain tissue, a procedure that can only be done at autopsy. A physician has to do the next best thing: rule out other causes before making a diagnosis. That's why so many tests have to be done, ranging from medical histories to psychiatric exams.

The patient usually sees the family doctor first. The doctor might perform an MRI (see next page), and then refer the patient to a specialist, such as a neurologist. The neurologist will then order the tests we are talking about. Some of the tests the patient may take are explained on the right. Note that not all professionals will order every exam listed here, nor will they necessarily do them in the order shown.

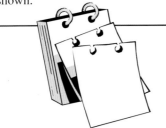

"It took weeks after the tests to find out that Daddy had Alzheimer's. Waiting was the one of the hardest things I have ever done."
—Beth

In these interviews, both family and patient are asked a series of questions that may require prior preparation. These may include:

- *What symptoms have you observed? When did you first notice them?*

- *Have the symptoms changed with time? How?*

- *Are their other medical conditions? Is the person taking medications?*

- *Do other family members have Alzheimer's? Past relatives?*

Part III | Mental Status Test

Assesses the patient's
- sense of time and place
- comprehension, memory
- ability to do simple calculations
- ability to complete mental exercises

Reason: This test examines brain function, just like a treadmill tests heart function. The doctor is careful to consider both background and education in evaluating the results.

Part II | Physical Exam

- Looks for presence of cardiac, respiratory, liver, kidney, thyroid disease.
- Evaluates the patient's nutritional status, blood pressure, pulse, other bodily functions.

Reason: Dementias can occur from many physical, non-Alzheimer's sources. These tests are designed to rule out other diseases that might also cause AD-like symptoms.

Part I | Medical History

- Interviews with patient
- Interviews with family members
- Interviews with patient and family members together

Reason: To gather background information on patient's current mental/physical states, history of previous illnesses, familial illnesses, assessment of daily functioning.

• EEG stands for electroencephalograph, a machine that measures the electrical activity of the brain. Other tests may be used in the exam as well, including:

• CT (computerized tomography), a procedure that examines brain tissue via X-rays. It is used to detect the presence of tumors, strokes, blood clots, etc.

• MRI (magnetic resonance imaging) is a procedure capable of detecting anomalies deep within the brain.

• Experimental techniques. Other procedures, while still in the research stage, may be employed during the exam. These could include PET (positron emission tomography) scans, which display areas of brain activity and SPECT (single photon emission computed tomography) scans, which display how blood circulates throughout the brain.

Part IV — Neurological Exam

Examines the nervous system. The doctor looks for evidence of previous strokes, parkinsonism, brain tumors, other disorders known to affect memory and thinking.

Reason: This series of tests attempts to further rule out other non-Alzheimer's disorders which might be causing the patient's symptoms.

Part V — Laboratory Tests

These tests assess blood chemistry and other bodily functions. Used to detect anemia, kidney and liver disorders, diabetes, levels of various vitamins, such as B_{12}, and folic acid.

Reason: These tests complement the physical and neurological exams, providing further hints as to the presence or absence of AD. A doctor may also order a test to detect abnormal brain wave activity (EEG).

Part VI — Psychiatric Exam

A psychiatric evaluation can rule out the presence of depression, which can create a memory loss similar to AD-associated dementia. Other exams evaluate reasoning, writing, vision-motor coordination, the ability to express ideas, etc. (these can provide more in-depth information than the mental status exam.) The tests may take several hours to complete, and may involve interviews as well as written examinations.

DIAGNOSIS

THE DIAGNOSIS

Once all the tests are done, the results will be evaluated and an opinion will be issued. The results generally fall into one of three categories, listed below. They are often communicated by a phone call from the family physician or diagnostic team.

• NOT ALZHEIMER'S

This conclusion is reached if the tests point to another cause. The exams may have uncovered evidence of a stroke, for example, or altered levels of a biochemical like thyroid hormone (which can cause a dementia that looks similar to AD).

• POSSIBLY ALZHEIMER'S

This conclusion occurs when the symptoms the patient is experiencing are atypical, but no other physical explanation is found. Something appears definitely to be wrong with the person, but no underlying explanation exists for the behavior other than AD.

• PROBABLY ALZHEIMER'S

This conclusion occurs when all the test results appear to be consistent with an AD profile, and no other causes for the symptoms are found. While this is truly a "ruling out" process, physicians can be 80% to 90% certain of their diagnosis when the proper tests are performed.

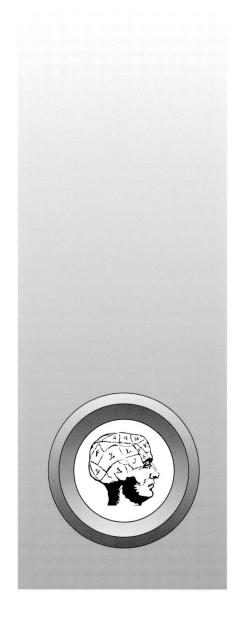

CHAPTER
TWO

*What Alzheimer's
looks like*

The outward signs of Alzheimer's disease

The brain is the seat of human behavior and mood. When diseases such as Alzheimer's destroy brain cells, changes in conduct and disposition can be expected.

The last chapter served as a general introduction to Alzheimer's disease, moving from prehistory to twentieth-century testing protocols. The goal of this chapter is to get a little more specific, characterizing in greater detail some of the outward manifestations of Alzheimer's disease. We will specifically examine behavior, mood, and medical problems people with AD commonly experience. This explanation will be clearer, however, if we first discuss a few basic facts about the human brain and its involvement in our actions and moods.

A COMPARTMENTALIZED HEAD

To truly understand how AD influences behavior, it must be realized that the brain is not a simple, single-purpose organ. Rather, it is a complex, mysterious, barely understood group of nerve cells, called *neurons*, divided into discrete regions. Different functions are assigned to different areas within the brain. There is a region of the brain for example, whose nerve cells allow us to speak. There is another area of the brain whose nerve cells allow us to see. These areas are connected by still other nerve cells whose job is to communicate information between saying and seeing. If that connection were ever broken, we could *see* something but might not be able to *say* what it is. The diagram on the right shows some of the areas of the brain and their assigned functions.

GRADUAL DESTRUCTION

Alzheimer's, as we have discussed, is a disease that kills nerve cells throughout this complex, regionalized brain. Nearly every area can be affected by the disorder, and neurons throughout the brain are destroyed in a gradual, cumulative fashion. Not only is the brain damaged slowly, it is also damaged unevenly. That's why a construction worker may still know how to drive a dump truck, but may not remember his wife's name. When a person with Alzheimer's does something strange or odd, it is because a part of the brain is no longer working correctly. Since other regions of the brain may be functioning normally, this can sometimes be difficult to believe.

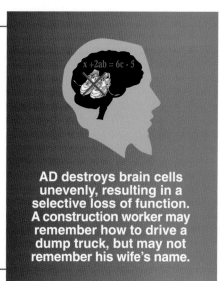

AD destroys brain cells unevenly, resulting in a selective loss of function. A construction worker may remember how to drive a dump truck, but may not remember his wife's name.

BEHAVIORS AND FEELINGS

Obviously, this multi-compartmentalized brain is the seat of everything in the human experience, including human behavior and mood. Not surprisingly, people with Alzheimer's disease can undergo dramatic changes in personality and disposition as their brains deteriorate. They may feel worried, lost, confused, anxious, and vulnerable. They may wander endlessly around the house or feel "the Mafia" is after them (about one-third, in fact, become mentally deranged). Some changes in behavior and disposition may be "normal" feelings of a panicked person reacting to a world slipping from his control. And even though such reactions do not have a basis in the reality of the caregiver, they are frighteningly real in the brain-damaged world of the person with Alzheimer's disease.

Each region of the brain has a specific function.

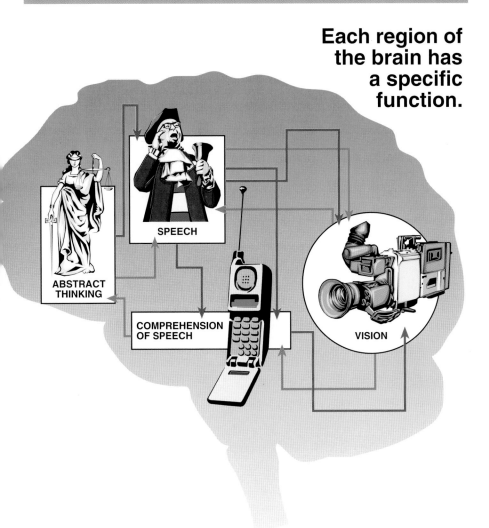

ABSTRACT THINKING

SPEECH

COMPREHENSION OF SPEECH

VISION

MEDICAL PROBLEMS

Besides mood changes, a person with Alzheimer's disease experiences certain medical problems. These include the normal kinds of illnesses we all experience from time to time. Also, medical problems exist that appear to be related specifically to Alzheimer's nerve damage. Uncle Ralph may become increasingly clumsy, falling out of bed, for example, cutting himself, perhaps breaking a bone. Because his or her brain is increasingly incapacitated, a confused person may not always be able to tell a caregiver what is wrong and, as such, the condition worsens.

A WORD ABOUT THE CHANGES

The relationship between this complicated brain, Alzheimer's disease, and behavior is direct, no matter whether we discuss behavior, mood, or medical issues: if certain areas of the brain get damaged, the function those areas normally supervise will be altered. This is the natural consequent of having Alzheimer's disease, *and such changes are not something the person can do anything about.* It can sometimes be easy to think that the afflicted person is doing something deliberately, especially if the behavior or mood change is obnoxious. But because the brain itself is being damaged, those behaviors are increasingly out of the control of the afflicted person.

> **Alzheimer's is not a fault. It is a disease.**

Behavior problems: Part 1

We begin our examination of AD's outward signs by discussing memory loss and the behavior problems that can arise from it.

The memory loss of Alzheimer's disease is very different from the loss due to normal aging. Deterioration due to AD can lead to redundant questioning, loss of precious items, shoplifting, seemingly endless repetition of certain actions, and so on. Behavior problems that occur with such losses are described below.

HIDING THE LOSS

People with AD sometimes attempt to conceal their loss of recall, especially in the early stages of the disease. Different people will react to their deficit in different ways, of course. But because the social skills and personalities of people with AD can remain intact for a long time, some may become quite adept at masking their declining abilities, even from loved ones.

REPETITION

Some manifestations of memory loss cannot be easily concealed. People with AD may ask the same question over and over again, for example. They may have no recollection of asking the question previously, and may be quite startled by an impatient response from the listener. Repetitious questioning may also be a symptom of anxiety and insecurity, based on the perception of an increasingly unstable world.

TAKING THINGS

People with Alzheimer's may take things that are not their own. Aunt Mary may shoplift because she simply forgets to pay for an item. She may not even realize she is in a store. Mary may even get mad at the sales clerk, accusing him of stealing her money. At home, a person with AD may take something from the neighbors and not return it. She may even accuse the neighbors of stealing the object if they attempt to reclaim it.

9/21/87

For the fifth time in a row Daddy said, "Of course I know that." He got angry at me for trying to explain to him exactly where to put the house keys, and now he was snapping back. But he didn't know where to put them. I found them once in my bedroom, once in the bath. I even found them in the refrigerator!

11/12/87

I have stopped asking Dr. Kramer to come by. Daddy keeps asking him how he's doing, and if he'd like some coffee. Kramer says he's doing fine, and that he already has a cup of coffee. Five minutes later Daddy asks him the same questions, even though Kramer's holding a half-full coffee cup. Kramer says he'd still like to visit.

12/16/87

Bill said that it was the last time he would take Daddy to the zoo. Daddy actually grabbed a duck and tried to take it home. Said it was Mom's Christmas present. The zoo people tried to take the bird from Daddy and he screamed so loud they kicked Daddy and Bill out. I don't think Bill has to worry about a return trip.

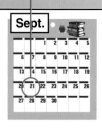

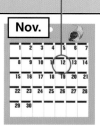

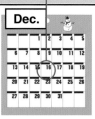

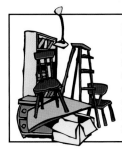

RUMMAGING BEHAVIOR

People with Alzheimer's disease sometimes rifle through their closets and dresser drawers. They may throw everything out, or attempt to rearrange the objects they find. This behavior can occur for a variety of reasons, including looking for a lost object (see below) but, invariably, they make a mess. This can be even more frustrating when the afflicted person starts to rummage through *other* people's closets and dresser drawers.

LOSING AND HIDING THINGS

Another sign of memory loss involves a person putting something down and then forgetting where he or she put it. Or consistently putting an object in a place where it does not belong. Some people with AD will hoard or collect things, and then forget the location of their stash. Because they truly don't remember, it may be futile to ask the person where the object is.

NUDITY AND SEXUAL BEHAVIOR

People with Alzheimer's disease do not always follow appropriate social conventions for clothing and sexual behavior. They may expose their genitals in public. They may fondle themselves, or repeat behaviors such as unzipping and zipping their trousers. It is a myth, however, that Alzheimer's patients will develop inappropriate sexual behaviors like child molestation or exhibitionism. Accidental self-exposure or masturbation may occur, but Alzheimer's seldom leads to criminal sexual activity.

> **It is a myth that Alzheimer's patients will develop sexual behaviors such as child molestation or exhibitionism.**

2/21/88

*I've given up trying to find quarters for downtown parking. I used to keep them in our spare-change jar, but the jar is now **always** empty. Amy says she overheard Daddy counting something in his room, and his door was closed. There was a clinking sound, she said, so I think I know where all the spare change is going.*

6/21/88

Bill was over to the house yesterday, right at the hottest part of the day. He came in through the alley and found Daddy sitting on the deck lounge, buck naked, in plain view of our neighbors. He was listening to Beethoven's Fifth Symphony. Bill said hi to Daddy and then ran into the house to find me. We found some old swim trunks and asked him to put them on. Daddy refused, saying it was too hot.

It is clear from these descriptions that memory loss can lead to severe disruptions in daily life, both for the caregiver and for the person with AD. These behaviors occur because areas in the brain responsible for memory are losing conections to other regions. Or the nerve cells holding the memories themselves are being destroyed. This damage has consequences that lead to other problems as well, such as distractibility and random wandering. These problems, and other issues like them, are discussed on the next page.

Feb.

	1	2	3	4	5	6
7	8	9	10	11	12	13
14	15	16	17	18	19	20
21	22	23	24	25	26	27
28	29					

June

			1	2	3	4
5	6	7	8	9	10	11
12	13	14	15	16	17	18
19	20	21	22	23	24	25
26	27	28	29	30		

Behavior problems: Part II

7/5/88

Daddy left the house for the third time this week. Only this time he found a shopping bag and put his church suit in it. I went running down our busy street after him, yelling at the top of my voice. Thank God he stopped where he was and waited for me! He said he was going back to Nebraska to see Grampa and Gramma, and wanted to know if I would come along.

WANDERING

Beth experienced with her father a common behavior associated with Alzheimer's disease, a seemingly inexplicable desire to wander. Sometimes the person will try to leave their living situation, even if it means wandering onto a busy intersection. Other times the afflicted person will drift from room to room. The wandering can change complexion and become an agitated, repetitive pacing. And it can happen any time of the day or night. The reason for such behavior is not well understood, though in some instances a purpose appears discernible. Some reasons wandering may occur are outlined below.

Getting lost

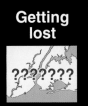

A person with AD may suddenly not know where she is. A grandmother may get up at night to go to the bathroom, and then forget where her bedroom is. She then spends the rest of the night wandering around the house, trying to find her sleeping quarters. Or she may become separated from a caregiver in a department store, and get lost trying to find her way back.

Orienting

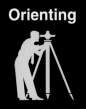

Wandering increases for some individuals when their living situation changes. The grandmother may begin a day care program, for example, or move with her family to a new living arrangement. She may wander for hours inspecting the new environment. Or she may not understand a move has occurred, and run around in a frantic search for her former house. This behavior is very common in nursing homes.

Expressing

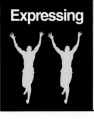

Wandering sometimes appears to represent an effort to say something. The person may feel a general sense of disorientation, attempting a remedy by looking for something familiar. Beth's dad, for example, was trying to get back to his childhood home, which may have symbolized for him feelings of security, stability, and friendship.

Sometimes wandering doesn't appear to have a reason. Seemingly incomprehensible pacing, determined and agitated, may have no other explanation than brain damage.

SOME WANDERING MAY BE EXPLAINED ONLY BY BRAIN DAMAGE

A person may persistently try to escape from a living situation, running from something that no one else can see. An afflicted uncle may get up in the middle of the night and think it is late evening, turning on the television, cooking the evening dinner. Though some kinds of wandering appear to have a purpose, other kinds remain inexplicable and undefined.

Inability to focus

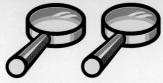

An often-overlooked characteristic of our brains is the ability to filter out and prioritize external inputs in the course of accomplishing a specific goal. For example, the doorbell might be ringing while you are putting on a shirt. Your brain allows you to prioritize this input: you first finish dressing and then answer the door. The brain of a person with AD can lose this ability to filter and prioritize. A grandfather might very well answer the door even though he hasn't finished dressing. He can be easily distracted simply because the ability to focus and organize inputs is slipping away from him.

THE NOT-SO-VISIBLE TALENTS OF THE BRAIN

It is clear from the previous examples that brain damage can be quite selective in a person with AD. These lesions—or sites of damage —shed light on the normal functioning of the brain as well, revealing specific areas controlling orientation and location. When such areas are damaged, we lose whatever abilities they supervised. These examples also show that the damage does not occur in an emotional vacuum; a person with Alzheimer's can react with just as much surprise and pain at the loss of ability as an unaffected loved one.

Our brains perform a number of functions that are not so obvious. That does not make them immune, however, from the ravages of Alzheimer's. Two such inconspicuous functions have to do with a) prioritizing and b) shifting gears.

Repetitious actions

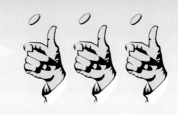

Related to prioritizing, another talent of the brain is the ability to shift gears from one task to another. This faculty might seem so obvious as to be not worth mentioning. But people with Alzheimer's disease can lose the ability and, as a result, endlessly repeat certain actions. For example, they might wash one side of their face, and when finished, immediately wash the same side. Or they might pace around in a circle for hours on end. Their brain appears to be "stuck" at some level, and they are unable to change patterns. Consequently, they repeat the same behavior over and over again.

Mood problems: Part I

People with Alzheimer's disease exhibit not only changes in behavior, but also alterations in mood and disposition. Some of these changes are summarized below.

There are many reasons people with Alzheimer's experience alterations in mood, ranging from brain damage to reactions to fading capabilities. We will discuss some specific changes and also some of the reasons why they may occur. Those reasons may be more apparent, however, if we first consider the world into which the confused person is plunged.

A TOPSY-TURVY PERSPECTIVE

As you know, the person with AD exists in a world that seems to be increasingly out of control. He is not going crazy, however. He is losing specific mental abilities that he used to take for granted, an event that can deeply affect a person's mood. Each minute of his life may consist of "starting over" with no memory of previous events. In this topsy-turvy world, familiar objects disappear without explanation. The immediate environment, just moments before filled with loved ones, now is populated only with strangers. His brain can no longer put information together in proper order; conversations cease to make sense, explanations are not remembered, people seem hostile without rhyme or reason. Such perceptions can lead to an almost continuous state of anxiety, irritability, paranoia, and depression. Considering all that an Alzheimer's patient must endure, it is small wonder that people with the disease often undergo changes in mood or disposition.

> **People with Alzheimer's are not going crazy; they are losing specific mental abilities they once took for granted.**

Specific mood changes

ANXIETY

It is very easy for a confused person to become worried and upset on a regular basis. This can be frustrating because the person may not be able to tell you why he or she is so anxious. Joan may be dimly aware she constantly "screw things up," feels powerless to do anything about it, and is anxious and worried most of the day.

IRRITABILITY

A person with AD may turn testy and contentious. She may get suddenly angry as the caregiver attempts to assist her with some task. She might throw things around the room, lash out at the caregiver verbally, even attempt to hit the caregiver.

DEPRESSION

The confused person may become depressed. There is a certain logic in suggesting that a person with AD may feel despondent because of the disease. But not all people with Alzheimer's are aware that something is wrong. Fortunately, Alzheimer's patients respond well to treatment for depression whether or not there is an awareness of the disease.

A STUDY IN PARANOIA

Some people with Alzheimer's disease become suspicious and exhibit paranoid behavior. Below is the transcript of a conversation Beth had with her father during an evening meal.

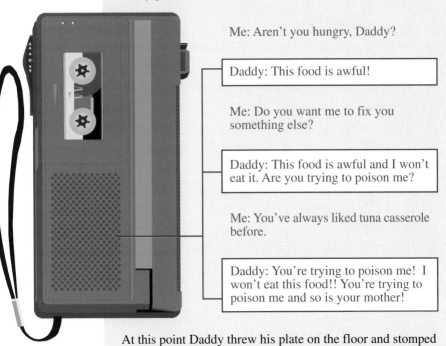

I tape-recorded a conversation I had with Daddy at the dinner table last night. I made his favorite dinner for him, and he barely picked at it.

Me: Aren't you hungry, Daddy?

Daddy: This food is awful!

Me: Do you want me to fix you something else?

Daddy: This food is awful and I won't eat it. Are you trying to poison me?

Me: You've always liked tuna casserole before.

Daddy: You're trying to poison me! I won't eat this food!! You're trying to poison me and so is your mother!

At this point Daddy threw his plate on the floor and stomped off to the bedroom. This was the second time this week he threw something off the table.

The conversation Beth recorded underscores a distressing fact: a confused person can become unreasonably suspicious, even paranoid. The person may develop an unshakable feeling that someone is out to get him. He may feel that someone is constantly stealing from him. Some of the reasons for this change in mood are outlined below:

MISINTERPRETATION. A confused person may consistently misjudge his environment. Uncle Erik may hear the sound of a fire siren, for example, and think it is a police wagon, coming to take him away. Hazel may hear very poorly, and interpret sounds as people whispering about her behind her back.

RECOGNITION FAILURE. Sometimes Alzheimer's causes the brain to lose links to previously familiar information. Mr. Petrie might say to his wife: "Who are you? Where is my wife? Why are you in my apartment?" Mr. Petrie actually retains a memory of his wife, but no can longer link that memory to what he sees with his eyes. As a result, he becomes fearful and paranoid of even familiar people in his living environment.

DELUSIONS. Confused people sometimes suffer delusions, untrue ideas or interpretations of ideas that have no basis in fact. People with Alzheimer's may feel gang members—or the Internal Revenue Service—is after them, or that someone is stealing their money. Though this is undoubtedly related to certain kinds of brain damage, no one really understands why this behavior is so common in people with AD.

Mood problems: Part II

6/13/88

Amy had Daddy the whole afternoon, which is some kind of record. Poor thing. He was in command mode, just like when he'd come home after a bad day at work. But this was awful. He shouted at Amy to turn the heat down in her apartment. Then he shouted at Amy to get him the newspaper. Five minutes later, he shouted at her to take the newspaper away and turn the heat up. This went on the whole afternoon. The last straw came when he shouted at Amy to get him a copy of *Light in August*, Daddy's favorite William Faulkner book. Amy doesn't even know who William Faulkner is! When Daddy went into a tantrum, she dumped him back on my doorstep and then took off. I only found out about this after I phoned her and did my own yelling. Was she in a bad mood!

A person with Alzheimer's disease can sometimes become very demanding. As in the excerpt above, this behavior may seem unreasonable—especially if the person is fully capable of performing the task he is requesting. It can be hard not to think of "Daddy" as being anything but self-centered, especially if he shows no other significant impairment from the disease.

Sometimes the demanding behavior signifies a loved one's growing fear of an unstable environment. Aunt Martha may no longer understand that her son is still in the house when he leaves the living room; instead she may feel he has just disappeared. Making demands of him may reassure her that her son is still around. The more demands made, the more she is reassured of his presence.

TENACIOUS DEPENDENCY

A mood problem that may also be associated with anxiety is emotional dependency, which can manifest itself in a clinging, sometimes desperate behavior. The person with AD may follow his caregiver around persistently, even from one room to the next. He may become anxious and irritable if his caregiver leaves him for just a minute. The caregiver may not even be able to go to the bathroom, or take a shower, without the loved one opening the door and following inside.

> **The caregiver may represent the only security the loved one has left in his confusing world.**

This behavior may be related to the same fearful perceptions as the demanding behavior. The caregiver may represent the only security the loved one has left in his confusing world. If he cannot rely on himself to stabilize his environment, he may cling tightly to the one who can.

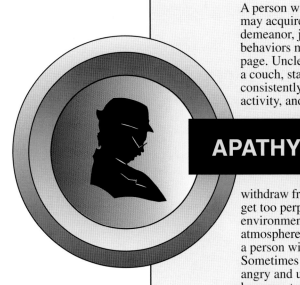

A person with Alzheimer's disease may acquire an apathetic and passive demeanor, just the opposite of the behaviors mentioned on the previous page. Uncle Gregory may just sit on a couch, staring at his lap. He may consistently refuse to engage in any activity, and become upset when his brother asks him to come outside. Such listlessness may reflect a confused person's need to withdraw from the world when things get too perplexing. If the amount of environmental stimuli is reduced, the atmosphere may seem more stable to a person with Alzheimer's disease. Sometimes the person may become angry and upset if the situation becomes too loud or action-filled.

APATHY

LOOSE CONNECTIONS

Some of these changes in personality have *no* logical or emotional explanation. They are simply due to an insidious loss of nerve cells. Caregivers often can become frustrated with their loved ones, trying to reason with them, hoping that they will change. But Alzheimer's is a disease of the brain, not a variable emotional state. As such, the person will never get better. They may change the way they manifest their symptoms (see below) but Alzheimer's is defined as a progressive and permanent destruction of nerve cells.

Another reason can make it difficult to accept that a loved one is brain-damaged. Sometimes a person with Alzheimer's disease appears to actually regain functions previously lost. Especially in the early stages, they may even have good days, when they seem more like themselves. Then for some inexplicable reason, they revert to their more dysfunctional pattern. It is a little bit like a loose connection between a lamp and an electrical outlet. Sometimes there are flickers of light, and sometimes there is only darkness. We do not know why the brain acts like this. But these intermittent changes can sometimes be deceptive—even cruel—fooling a caregiver into thinking a loved one is actually getting better.

Medical problems and Alzheimer's disease: Part I

Though their behaviors and moods may change, people with AD have normal bodies that require ordinary medical attention, just like anyone else. The problem is, they can't always tell you what is wrong.

Whether the cause is major or minor, it is a fact of life that humans require medical attention. While Alzheimer's itself does not directly cause pain, the disease does not exempt the patient from everyday illnesses and accidents. Where a problem may exist with AD is in the loved one's ability to communicate what is wrong. Though the patient may feel intense discomfort, the only sign a caregiver may encounter is some kind of change in mood or behavior (most confusing of all, such change may not seem related to anything medical). Another difficulty with AD is that the person may not remember if he or she had, say, an accident. Inconspicuous injury may go unnoticed for long periods of time.

It is of course important to understand the individual signs a person with AD may be attempting to communicate regarding their health. Listed on this page are some common warning signs Alzheimer's

These changes ...

- a worsening disposition
- refusal to do certain things
- increased restlessness
- worsening of specific behaviors
- moaning or shouting
- refusal to eat or drink

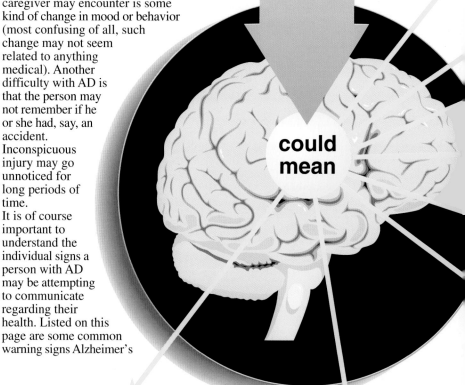

could mean

PRESSURE SORES

Sometimes called bedsores, these painful ulcers develop on the skin when someone sits or lies down for long periods of time. They can also occur because of ill-fitting clothing or lack of adequate nutrition.

DEHYDRATION

People with AD sometimes forget to drink. Ensuring proper hydration is especially important if the loved one has had diarrhea, diabetes or has been vomiting.

CONSTIPATION

Alzheimer's patients may be oblivious as to whether or not they have regular bowel movements. They may not realize that the discomfort they feel is due to constipation.

PNEUMONIA

Pneumonia is an infection of the lungs caused by bacteria and viruses. A frequent complication of AD, its presence can be difficult to detect. Delirium is sometimes the earliest symptom.

BRUISES, SCRAPES AND BROKEN BONES

A person with Alzheimer's disease may have a greater tendency to be clumsy. It may be easy for her to trip, fall off a chair, run into things, bruise or cut herself. Since a person with AD tends to be older, she has more fragile bones, drier and thinnner skin. As a result, she has a greater tendency to suffer more serious injuries from minor falls or abrasions. This is made worse if she forgets she has fallen, or refuses to tell you she is in pain.

DENTAL PROBLEMS

Cavities, sores, gum and mouth abscesses occur frequently with Alzheimer's patients, especially if the afflicted person was taking care of himself. Finding what is wrong can be made more difficult because a person with AD may not allow a caregiver to look in his mouth.

SIDE EFFECTS

Loved ones may be taking medications for conditions unrelated to their Alzheimer's. These medicines, while useful, may also have unwanted side effects that cause irritation and discomfort. The patient with Alzheimer's may not always be able to articulate the impact of these side effects on their well-being.

PROBLEMS WITH VISION

People with Alzheimer's sometimes appear to be going blind. They bump into familiar objects, become lost in dim light, misplace valuable things. The problem of vision in AD patients is complicated by several issues. Most loved ones with Alzheimer's are older, for example, so their vision is quite naturally changing (they may become farsighted, they may adjust more slowly to changing light conditions, cataracts may be forming, and so on). In dim light, things are harder to see under normal circumstances. For a person with Alzheimer's this difficulty can be traumatic; dawn and dusk may become the most confusing parts of the day. Moreover, because of brain impairment, a loved one might see perfectly, but lose the ability to comprehend what is being visualized. For example, they may interpret a table as "not really being there" and attempt to walk right through it.

Medical problems: Part II

3/2/91
I have been noticing for the past few weeks that Daddy is getting slower and slower—especially when he walks. I took him out for a stroll a couple of days ago. He lifted his feet high into the air at each step, almost like he was stepping over a puddle. I was *so* embarrassed! For a long time now he has been holding on to doors and chairs when he moves around the house. I've even seen him standing in the hall, grabbing at nothing, like he was shadowboxing or something.

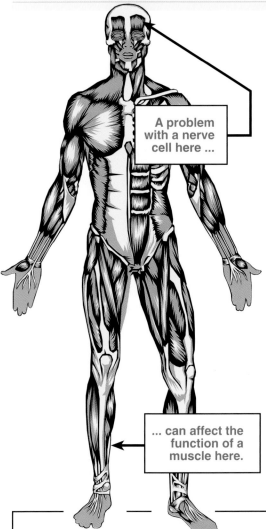

A problem with a nerve cell here ...

... can affect the function of a muscle here.

MOTOR PROBLEMS

Some of the behavior that Beth describes above illustrates a familiar medical issue: Alzheimer's disease can affect a person's physical ability to move. As described on the previous pages, the person may become awkward, bumping into things. He may have difficulty getting out of bed. The person with AD may become bent or develop a stooping posture, shuffling when he walks. Such developments are usually seen in the later stages of disease. Like Daddy, a person may even hallucinate (though this is a separate issue from the motor problems discussed here and will be dealt with later).

There are many non-Alzheimer's reasons why such conditions develop (the side effects of medications, for example). But, sadly, Alzheimer's disease is fully capable of attacking the part of the brain that controls muscles. Smaller steps and repeated falls may, after a period of years, result in a person's inability to stand up and move.

SPORADIC INVOLUNTARY MOVEMENTS

A person with AD sometimes develops rapid, jerking movements. These sudden motions may involve movement of the legs, arms, head, or upper body. Called *myoclonic jerks*, such involuntary "twitches" are different from seizures, which are repeated movements of the same muscle groups. Rather, myoclonic jerks are single motions of a limb, head, or other body part. No one knows why Alzheimer's patients experience these odd motions. And currently, there is no treatment for the condition.

INCONTINENCE

In addition to motor loss, Alzheimer's patients may lose their ability to control bowel and bladder function. This can be serious because wet or soiled clothing can very quickly lead to sores, rashes, and other skin irritations.

In the case of bladder malfunction, a person with AD may constantly wet herself. There are many medical reasons for urinary incontinence, including bladder infections, diabetes, weakening muscles in the bladder, and side effects of medications. This loss of control can occur in several patterns, each of which may indicate a different cause. Here are three:

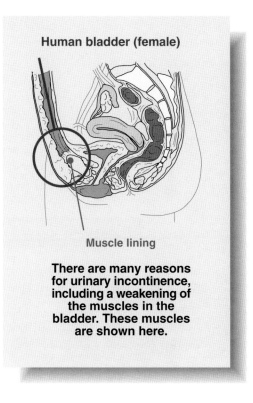

Human bladder (female)

Muscle lining

There are many reasons for urinary incontinence, including a weakening of the muscles in the bladder. These muscles are shown here.

• Leaking (especially if the patient is a woman, she may not really be emptying the bladder, but leaking when she coughs, sneezes, laughs or lifts something).

• Accidents that occurs only during certain times of the day (such as at night).

• Accidents that occurs on the way to the bathroom.

Losing control of bowel and bladder function may not mean incontinence for the Alzheimer's patient, however. Sometimes the loss is just a reflection of general confusion. A patient may express urinating needs in verbal forms which mean something else to the caregiver. Aunt Martha may ask to "walk the dog" when she needs to use the toilet, a cue the caregiver may not understand. Uncle Ralph may decide to urinate in the kitchen trash can; if he can't find it, he may simply wet his clothing when his bladder is full. Sometimes a familiar action may trigger incontinence. Every time a caregiver pulls down a patient's undershorts, for example, the patient may try to defecate. Confusion may occur simply because the patient has a memory that he moved his bowels every time he pulled down his briefs.

SUMMARY

In persons with AD, medical problems must be seen in the same understanding light as mood and behavior problems. Often it is a problem of communication. It is natural for unaffected individuals to complain and describe what is wrong with them. But because Alzheimer's attacks the brain, there is no guarantee that a person who is in need of attention will know how to get it. It can be a vicious circle, for as the brain deteriorates, the body loses more functions, becoming increasingly vulnerable. We will discuss in greater detail how to deal with such problems in the third section of this book.

When does death occur?

Regardless of mood, behavior, or medical problems, the end result of Alzheimer's disease is death. Perhaps surprisingly, when and how the end occurs is not easy to predict.

The sad fact of Alzheimer's is that it is progressively and unstoppably fatal. No one has ever successfully recovered to full health once diagnosed with AD. In the final stages of the disease, the brain has taken so much nerve damage that the body cannot cope. Death ensues.

While such gloomy facts are well-known, it is actually tricky to specify how AD causes human death. This is because very few people die directly from the disease. The end usually comes obliquely, from some common medical complication frequently associated with Alzheimer's. In an attempt to organize this ambiguity, medical professionals have adopted the concepts of *immediate cause* and *actual cause* of death for many diseases, including Alzheimer's. Here's an example of how it works:

Mr. Nolan, who has Alzheimer's disease, wanders out of the house and onto a busy street. He is struck by a passing taxicab, suffers massive head injuries and dies en route to the hospital.

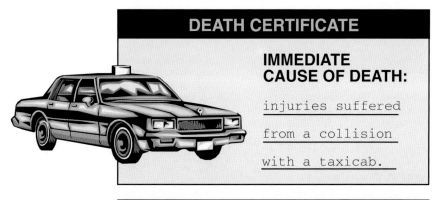

DEATH CERTIFICATE

IMMEDIATE CAUSE OF DEATH:

injuries suffered from a collision with a taxicab.

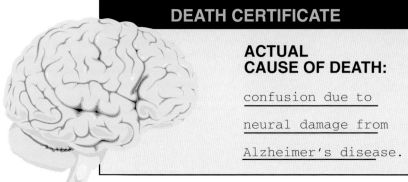

DEATH CERTIFICATE

ACTUAL CAUSE OF DEATH:

confusion due to neural damage from Alzheimer's disease.

Thus, even though technically Mr. Nolan died of head injuries in an auto accident, he might not have been on the street if he didn't have Alzheimer's. The actual cause of death is AD, regardless of the immediate cause.

Does this sound picky? In times past, death certificates often listed only immediate causes, which made life difficult for researchers trying to make meaningful studies of mortality and Alzheimer's. Fortunately, reporting practices have started to change, and more accurate statistics are becoming available. Some of these data are shown on the next page.

HOW DO MOST ALZHEIMER'S PATIENTS DIE?

The immediate cause of death for patients with Alzheimer's include accidental deaths (like Mr. Nolan's), infections, malnutrition and dehydration. There is some evidence to suggest that the level of mental impairment may have something to do with the kind of death experienced.

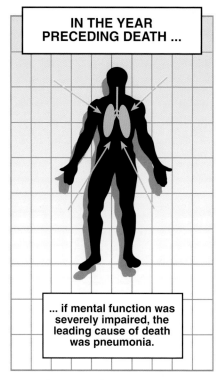

IN THE YEAR PRECEDING DEATH ...

... if mental function was severely impaired, the leading cause of death was pneumonia.

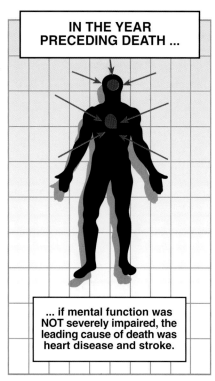

IN THE YEAR PRECEDING DEATH ...

... if mental function was NOT severely impaired, the leading cause of death was heart disease and stroke.

HOW LONG DOES IT TAKE TO DIE?

Regardless of the cause of death, the most agonizing question for the caregiver has to do with the length of time a loved one will suffer. The most useful calculation would be the time from when symptoms first appear until the person dies. It can be difficult, however, to accurately assess when Alzheimer's symptoms *really* started appearing versus the time a family member or friend noticed that something was actually wrong. (As we'll see on the next page, the average length of time between someone's noticing a symptom versus taking them to a physician for diagnosis is almost three years!) Nonetheless, one research group found that time until death depended upon the age of symptom onset, as shown below:

YEARS UNTIL DEATH ...

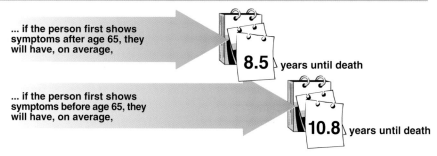

... if the person first shows symptoms after age 65, they will have, on average, **8.5** years until death

... if the person first shows symptoms before age 65, they will have, on average, **10.8** years until death

These researchers found that the younger the person was at symptom onset, the longer it took to die. It is important to realize that this is just one study, of course. Patients have been known to die in as little as three or as many as twenty years after symptoms were first discovered.

The course of the disease

The progression and time of death are different for each person afflicted with AD. Here's the history of the disease as experienced by Beth's father, compared to the national average.

As research methods improve we get a clearer picture of both the causes of death and the length of time before death ensues. Enough data exists that a national timeline can be constructed. On this page, we illustrate the disease progression of Beth's father, and show how his timeline compares with the U.S. profile.

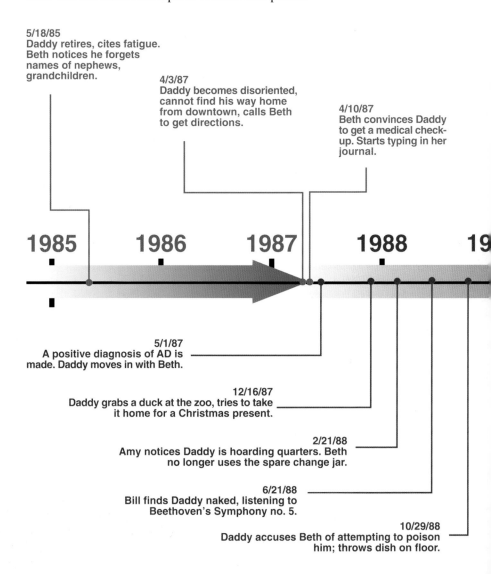

5/18/85
Daddy retires, cites fatigue. Beth notices he forgets names of nephews, grandchildren.

4/3/87
Daddy becomes disoriented, cannot find his way home from downtown, calls Beth to get directions.

4/10/87
Beth convinces Daddy to get a medical check-up. Starts typing in her journal.

1985   1986   1987   1988   19

5/1/87
A positive diagnosis of AD is made. Daddy moves in with Beth.

12/16/87
Daddy grabs a duck at the zoo, tries to take it home for a Christmas present.

2/21/88
Amy notices Daddy is hoarding quarters. Beth no longer uses the spare change jar.

6/21/88
Bill finds Daddy naked, listening to Beethoven's Symphony no. 5.

10/29/88
Daddy accuses Beth of attempting to poison him; throws dish on floor.

THE NATIONAL AVERAGE
Daddy's experience with Alzheimer's is similar to the national profile of AD in males over 65. Beth first noticed symptoms back in '85 when Daddy could not recall the names of his young relatives. At right is a comparison of Daddy's history, starting in '85, with the national average of persons over 65.

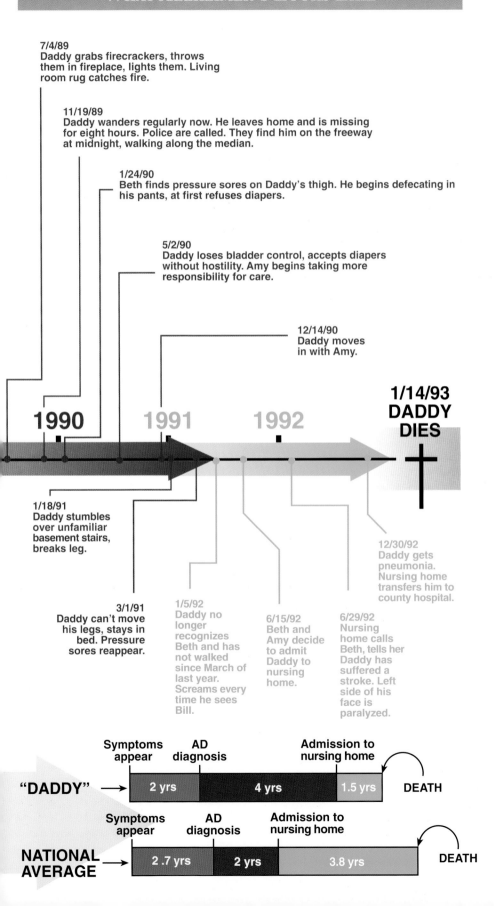

7/4/89
Daddy grabs firecrackers, throws them in fireplace, lights them. Living room rug catches fire.

11/19/89
Daddy wanders regularly now. He leaves home and is missing for eight hours. Police are called. They find him on the freeway at midnight, walking along the median.

1/24/90
Beth finds pressure sores on Daddy's thigh. He begins defecating in his pants, at first refuses diapers.

5/2/90
Daddy loses bladder control, accepts diapers without hostility. Amy begins taking more responsibility for care.

12/14/90
Daddy moves in with Amy.

1990 **1991** **1992**

1/14/93 DADDY DIES

1/18/91
Daddy stumbles over unfamiliar basement stairs, breaks leg.

12/30/92
Daddy gets pneumonia. Nursing home transfers him to county hospital.

3/1/91
Daddy can't move his legs, stays in bed. Pressure sores reappear.

1/5/92
Daddy no longer recognizes Beth and has not walked since March of last year. Screams every time he sees Bill.

6/15/92
Beth and Amy decide to admit Daddy to nursing home.

6/29/92
Nursing home calls Beth, tells her Daddy has suffered a stroke. Left side of his face is paralyzed.

Symptoms appear   AD diagnosis   Admission to nursing home

"DADDY" → | 2 yrs | 4 yrs | 1.5 yrs | DEATH

Symptoms appear   AD diagnosis   Admission to nursing home

NATIONAL AVERAGE → | 2.7 yrs | 2 yrs | 3.8 yrs | DEATH

why

discovering why Alzheimer's destroys the brain

- *Problems defining human memory*

- *What the brain looks like from the inside*

- *Where in the brain memory occurs*

- *What a nerve cell looks like*

- *How nerve cells talk to each other*

- *DNA and genes*

- *The types of Alzheimer's diseases*

- *Of plaques and Alzheimer's*

- *Of tangles and Alzheimer's*

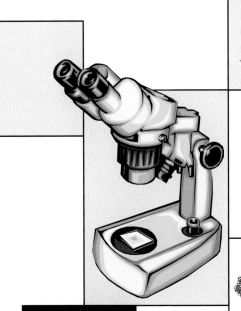

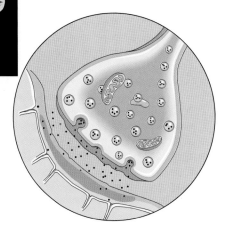

Introduction to section two

The goal of this section is to explain how Alzheimer's disease ravages the human brain. To accomplish the goal, we must address four basic topics in brain biology.

3/14/89

I give up trying to make sense of this thing. I just caught Daddy in the bathtub, splashing water over the floor like a two-year-old. He was a doctor, for God's sake! He used to operate on people! He spoke with words I will never understand and used to answer everyone's questions and *everybody* looked to him for advice. Now he can't even tie his shoe! How do I explain his behavior to his friends, or to what's left of his family? Like me?

The biology of Alzheimer's

The "why" questions Beth writes in her journal are asked by just about everyone who encounters Alzheimer's disease. Daddy might rattle off some complex medical fact from an old journal one minute, and then lose his way to the bathroom the next. Or he might integrate several memories at once; Daddy once tried to scrub for surgery in the kitchen sink just before dinner. Why does Alzheimer's do such a thing? What is it about damaged nerve cells and molecules that could turn functioning adults into seemingly helpless children?

The same questions that caused Beth such anguish have been asked by researchers for many years. In this section, we will attempt to answer some of them. To understand what is known about the "whys" of AD, we must review some basic biology of the brain and nerves. The first two chapters will cover basic biology of memory, brains, nerves, and molecules. The last chapter will talk about Alzheimer's. Here's a description of where we are going.

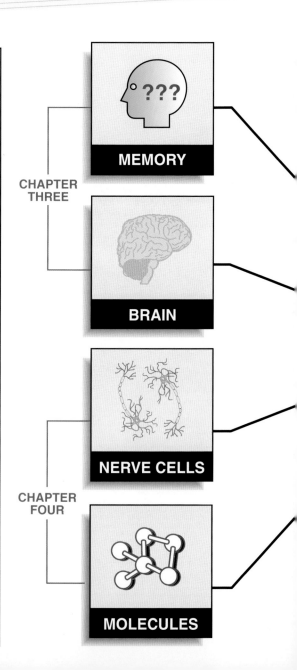

MEMORY

CHAPTER THREE

BRAIN

NERVE CELLS

CHAPTER FOUR

MOLECULES

MEMORY

Our first task is to understand how human memory works. Such background will give us better insights into what happens when memory is damaged. We will discover that this obvious human talent can be surprisingly difficult to define. There appear to be several kinds of memory systems in human brains, however, and we will take a look at several in this section.

BRAIN ANATOMY

Since Alzheimer's is a disease of brain tissue, we next enter into a discussion of brain anatomy. As previously mentioned, different regions of the brain appear to be responsible for different tasks. Because discrete functions are compartmentalized, a person with AD might lose one function yet be perfectly capable in other areas. Understanding how this works together can give us powerful clues into the sometimes baffling behavior of Alzheimer's patients.

NERVE CELLS

Our next task is to examine how the individual nerve cells work in our brains. Specifically, we will describe what neurons look like and how they are used to carry human thought. But not just to gain better insights into memory. The various regions of the brain have to communicate with each other in order for the organ to work properly. This communication, which can break down readily in Alzheimer's disease, is also facilitated by nerve cells. We will look at how this communication works.

MOLECULES

Some of most exciting research into Alzheimer's disease is also some of the most intimate, the tiny world of genes and the molecules they produce. To understand this knowledge, we must first discuss how genes become activated and how their dysfunction can lead to disease. Perhaps most importantly, we will obtain a background necessary to discuss a startling fact: that there is a genetic component to Alzheimer's disease, and that some of these genes appear to have been isolated.

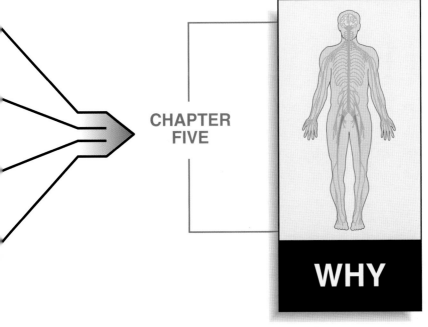

CHAPTER
FIVE

WHY

... Alzheimer's damages the brain

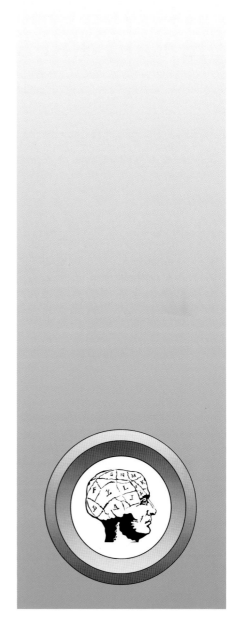

CHAPTER
THREE

*Memory and
the brain*

Problems defining memory: the long and short of it

Though memory can be difficult to define, researchers have attempted to conceptually organize its structure. Based on time of retention, memory can be divided into short and long components.

From the organizational chart on the previous pages, it is clear we are taking a "top down" approach to this background review, starting with very large concepts and moving to very tiny molecules. The first large concept we consider is the structure of memory.

A PROBLEM

We are all very familiar with the concept of memory. You can read this page because of memory, recollecting your experience with the English language, recalling individual phrases, sentences, words, even grammatical rules. Don't let that familiarity fool you, however. Even though we all have critical experiences with the process of memory, it can be difficult to describe what memory is, let alone define it. That's true especially if you are a scientist trying to make sense of memory from a research point of view. Here are some examples of why this difficulty exists:

More than one kind of memory?

Riding a bicycle is not the same as speaking a foreign language. Different systems of memory may be used to accomplish each skill.

In his healthy days, Beth's father was an avid cyclist. And because he was an immigrant (from Germany), he spoke several languages. It seems intuitively obvious, even though bicycling and language both require memory, that they are not the same recollection process. Language requires a person to use a word correctly, remembering its meaning and proper usages. Riding a bicycle requires remembering a complex series of muscle movements, all in coordination with a sense of balance, all reacting to a constantly changing terrain. Indeed, when Daddy became sick, he often could not remember the word for bicycle in either German or English. Yet he retained the ability to ride a bicycle until he became bedridden.

SO HOW IS MEMORY ORGANIZED?

In trying to organize these various talents, researchers have concluded that memory is not a unitary process. Instead, there appear to be multiple kinds of memory, each with different features, perhaps employing different parts of the brain to accomplish their goals Over the years, several models have been put forward to explain the structure of human memory.

DIVIDING MEMORY INTO PARTS

It is possible to divide our memory into several categories by looking at a timing event—specifically, examining how long we can retain pieces of information in our heads. Scientists have found that we possess several capacities for retaining bits of knowledge. Several of these are described below.

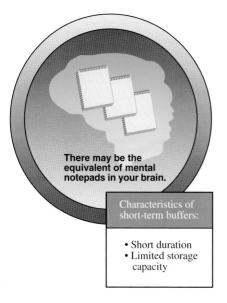

There may be the equivalent of mental notepads in your brain.

Characteristics of short-term buffers:

- Short duration
- Limited storage capacity

SHORT-TERM BUFFERS

One form of memory allows us to keep objects or events in mind for only short periods of time (usually measured in a time scale of seconds). It's as if there were small mental notepads inside our skulls. Scientists call these notepads *buffers*. Something may be "jotted down" in the buffers for a few moments, but quickly lost afterward. A short-term buffer, for example, is used when you find a number in a phone directory and dial it. You remember the phone number only for the length of time it takes you to grab the phone and punch in the numbers. But you quickly forget the numbers as the conversation begins. Different buffers appear to hold different types of information at the same time (sensory versus spatial versus language, for example). In addition to timing, the amount of information that a short-term buffer can hold at any one time appears to be limited.

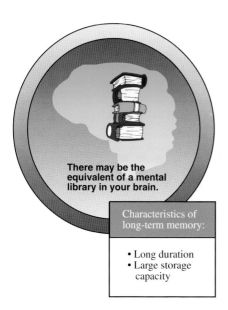

There may be the equivalent of a mental library in your brain.

Characteristics of long-term memory:

- Long duration
- Large storage capacity

LONG-TERM MEMORY

Our brains also have a capacity known as *long-term memory*, something very different from the mental notepad described above. Also called *secondary memory*, this form of remembering lasts much longer than a few seconds. Indeed, long-term memory can hold a piece of information for the duration of a person's life. Moreover, we seem to have an almost unlimited capacity to remember objects or events in long-term memory. You can think of long-term memory as a mental library; there are lots of books already on the shelves storing previously encountered information, and there are many empty shelves upon which to place new information as the years go by. How pieces of information can pass from short-term buffers to long-term memory is not well-understood.

WORKING MEMORY

Our brains also appear to have a type of memory that serves as an executive liaison between our short-term buffers and long-term storage. Called *working memory*, this extraordinary process manages information by looking in the short-term buffers, yet processing information dragged up from long-term memory at the same time. This kind of memory is useful for performing a wide range of tasks that require both buffers and more permanent storage (reading, for example, or even mental arithmetic).

Other types: how long-term memory may be organized

To explain certain learning behaviors, researchers have proposed subdivisions in long-term memory. Here are four commonly accepted categories.

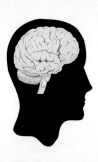

The vast and multifaceted nature of memory has not easily lent itself to a classification scheme upon which all researchers agree. Fortunately, the distinctions between short-term buffers and long-term memory have become clearer as the years roll by. Attempts have been made to further explain long-term memory by subdividing it into component parts.

Illustrated on these two pages is one classification scheme described in the research literature by a group of British researchers.* They agree that memory can be divided into short-term and long-term components. They further explain that long-term memory is itself subdivided into discrete categories.

When viewing the categories listed on these pages, it must be remembered that the distinctions between them are mostly conceptual. What does that mean? Classifications of memory are derived from observations of people in laboratory situations, and we have derived *concepts* of memory based on what has been observed. These categories do not come from looking at brain tissue and finding areas for specific types of recall. Most researchers use conceptual classifications as a framework for further experimentation and refinement of their ideas. That's why scientists don't always agree on the organization of human memory. It doesn't mean these categories are useless; the diversity simply reflects differences in the opinions of the researchers involved. As we'll see, areas of brain tissue have been found that appear to control at least some of these categories of memory.

* Fletcher, P.C., R.J. Dolan and C.D. Frith. 1995. The functional anatomy of memory. *Experientia* 51:1197-1207. See also related references at the end of this book.

1

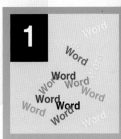

EXPLICIT

There is a class of memory known as *explicit memory*. It includes recollections that can willfully be brought to consciousness and expressed verbally. Suppose, for example, you are presented with a series of words, and then someone asks you to repeat the words you encountered. Such recall, brought to consciousness deliberately, is the hallmark of explicit memory.

IS THERE A CONNECTION BETWEEN SHORT- AND LONG-TERM MEMORY?

Yes, though no knows exactly how they are related. It is clear that the type of information being received by the listener plays a role in retention. Inputs having a greater relevance or significance to the person, such as those that create emotional arousal, have the best chance of being encoded into long-term memory. Exposure to meaningless information, regardless of the length of exposure, has the least chance of being retained.

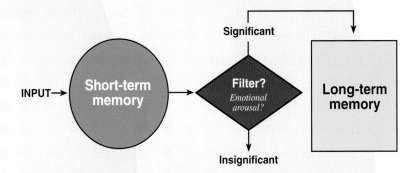

INPUT→ **Short-term memory** → **Filter?** *Emotional arousal?*

Significant → **Long-term memory**

Insignificant

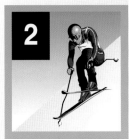

IMPLICIT

Another category, called *implicit memory*, is in direct contrast to the explicit variety. Implicit memory does not depend on explicit conscious recollection. Rather, this form of memory is non-intentional and accumulates quite slowly, through repetition and practice. The ability to perform a motor skill such as skiing —even if many years go by—is an example of implicit memory.

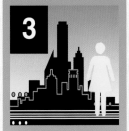

EPISODIC

Episodic memory is a form of recollection that has two components: First, it is autobiographical in context, which means the person is actively involved in whatever is going to be remembered. Secondly, this type of memory is episodic in context, which means the person recalls a specific occurrence in which he or she is involved. For example, a memory of New York might be episodic in that the person recalls experiencing her first Broadway show or her first visit to the Empire State Building.

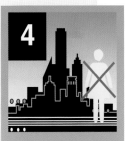

SEMANTIC

Semantic memory is just the opposite of episodic memory. This kind of recollection is not personalized, nor is it episodic in form. Semantic memory refers to factual knowledge used in the comprehension and structuring of symbols (both visual and verbal). The semantic memory of New York might be composed of the knowledge that the city is in the United States, is so many square miles in size, houses the headquarters of the United Nations and so on. It would not per se include the memory of the person's visit to the city.

Organization of memory and Alzheimer's disease

The various categories of memory can be organized into a flow chart, as below, to help us better understand patients with AD.

The categories of memory described on the previous page have been organized by the same researchers into a chart. Structurally, this graphic provides a convenient framework for helping us understand the behavior of patients with Alzheimer's disease. It must be remembered, however, that this framework is conceptual only; many important details about human memory have yet to be categorized.

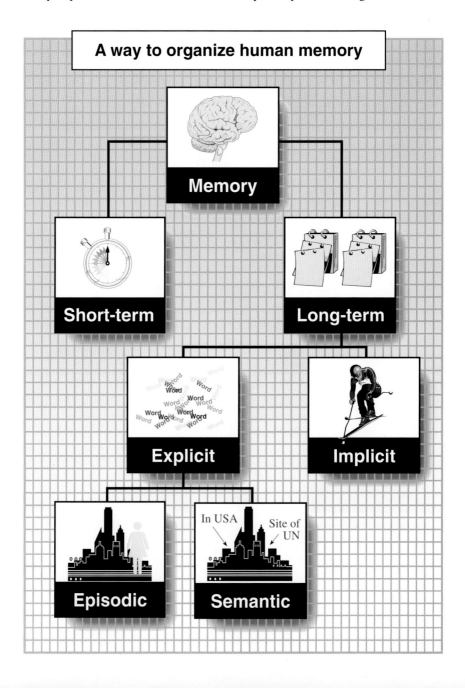

WHAT DOES THIS HAVE TO DO WITH ALZHEIMER'S?

Potentially, a lot. It is possible to understand the bizarre behaviors of Alzheimer's patients in terms of increasingly dysfunctional memory systems, like the system shown on the previous page. Below are descriptions of Alzheimer's behavior, taken from Beth's journal, and what may be occurring in Daddy's memory while the behavior takes place. At this point, such associations are entirely speculative (scientists who cannot agree on the categories will certainly not agree on links between them and a disease process). But the examples may be instructive. They may provide a way for caregivers to make sense of behaviors that might otherwise seem erratic and random. And they point to research directions scientists take as they seek to understand the links between behavior and memory.

Daddy kept asking who had come to the door yesterday. I told him it was his friend from the hospital, John. Daddy smiled and he asked me how John's two kids were doing. Not even five minutes later, Daddy wandered into the kitchen and asked me who was at the door yesterday. I told him who it was and then Daddy asked me the question about his kids *again*. Then a minute later, while I was putting some dishes away, he asked me one more time who came to the door yesterday.

Possible interpretation: Some form of Daddy's short-term memory was dysfunctional. His long-term memory seemed intact as far as his friend was concerned (he recognized John, knew he had children, and even how many). But Daddy could not recall Beth's answers to his questions, and so repeatedly asked them over and over again.

Today I had to re-teach Daddy how to use a knife and fork. I could tell he was hungry. When he asked me what was for lunch and I told him, he immediately went down to the kitchen and waited at the table. But when I served him the food, Daddy just stared at it with a blank look. I actually had to show Daddy how to use the utensils! He was real awkward, but after awhile Daddy got the hang of it and finished his lunch.

Possible interpretation: Daddy's short-term memory seemed to function, at least retaining the ability to remember that food would soon be served at lunch. But he lost a particular motor skill, the ability to use common tableware. Such skills are the province of implicit memory, and might indicate dysfunction in this memory category.

I took Daddy out for some exercise and got him to ride his bicycle. It was tough! Daddy didn't recognize me all morning. He kept batting me away and constantly asked where Beth was. Me! It took forever to get him off the bike and back into the house.

Possible interpretation: As Daddy retained the skill to ride his bicycle, some facet of implicit memory was working adequately. But there was definitely long-term memory loss, because Daddy no longer recognized Beth as his daughter.

These memory systems represent only one way to organize human memory. And there are more proposed memory categories than described here (we did not even mention the vital concepts of storage and retrieval, which can be helpful in distinguishing Alzheimer's from diseases like Parkinson's). As research progresses, however, we will better understand which memory systems reflect biological reality and which were just educated guesses. In a few cases, areas in the brain have been isolated that appear to govern specific parts of the human memory just discussed. To understand this research (and its impact on our understanding of AD) we will need to review a few facts about the anatomy of our brains.

What the brain looks like

The human brain is divided into a number of discrete regions. Both structurally and functionally the organ is highly compartmentalized.

The categories of memory, whichever ones turn out to be true, are all tucked within the most complex—and talented—object on earth. Composed of billions of nerve cells, our brains gives us our intelligence, our ability to sense our surroundings, our very identities. With so many important functions under its control, it is small wonder that so many things go wrong when the brain is damaged. To understand why Alzheimer's can be so crippling, we need to address some organizational features of the brain, and then review some of its basic anatomy. We begin by discussing three fundamental facts.

#1) THE BRAIN IS COMPARTMENTALIZED

The human brain is not a homogenous, uniform thinking network. Rather, the brain consists of individual structures that appear to perform, in many cases, specific tasks. There are regions responsible for vision, for speaking, for certain types of reasoning, even for feeling emotions such as love and rage. There are places where we store memories of pictures, and these seem to be different from the places where we store the words that describe the pictures. Just how meticulous this compartmentation is has only recently begun to be appreciated.

#2) THESE COMPARTMENTS ARE INTERCONNECTED

Though specific regions of the brain have discrete job assignments, an unbelievably complex web of nerve cells interconnects all of them. Such organization can be likened to superhighway systems linking various cities together. Some of these highways, composed of individual nerve cells, have been mapped. The routes they describe exhibit the same complexity of organization. In many cases, the highways themselves perform the specific function (as if the country road connecting two dairies actually produced the milk!). This blurs the distinction between connectors and the "regions" they serve.

#3) INDIVIDUAL COMPARTMENTS CAN BE DESTROYED

And so can their connections. Because specific regions are responsible for individual tasks, when the region is destroyed, so is the ability to perform that task. In Alzheimer's disease, some regions of the brain are rendered dysfunctional before other areas. This means that a person like Beth's father may be able to perform one task, like suturing a wound, yet be unable to identify common food items in a grocery store.

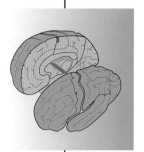

Keeping the idea of compartmentation in mind, we are ready to discuss some brain anatomy.

Consider the drawing on the left. You can see that, from an overall perspective, the brain is like a small watermelon split down the middle. As is true with most brain structures, those two halves of the brain are very well connected. Superhighways of nerve cells, collectively termed the *corpus callosum*, traverse them, allowing communication between the halves.

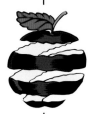

THE HEMISPHERES HAVE A COVERING

The surfaces of the brain's hemispheres (actually, the cerebral hemispheres) are blanketed with a thin coating of nerve cells called the *cortex*. You can think of the cortex covering a brain the same way you might think of the skin covering an apple. The cortex is responsible for tasks that include, among other things, interpreting sensory information and creating and controlling certain emotional and intellectual processes (see drawing below).

The halves of the brain can be further subdivided into specific regions.

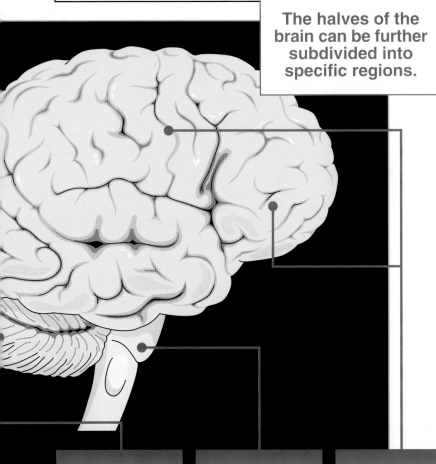

The first region

The region sitting directly at the back of the brain is called the *cerebellum*. It is responsible for motor functions, such as coordinating movement, maintenance of posture, and balance.

The second region

The *medulla* is the part of the brain that joins it to the spinal column. It regulates functions such as blood pressure, heart rate, and respiration.

The third region

The largest part of the brain is the *cerebrum*, and the cortex that overlays it the *cerebral cortex*. The functions of this vast area are complex and will be discussed later.

Where does memory occur?

The areas that control human memory are beginning to be mapped. This map is being refined by examining people who have undergone strokes.

We have spent the past few pages discussing both the structure of human memory and the structure of human brains. Is it possible to associate the two? Is there evidence that certain brain structures mediate certain kinds of memory? In some cases, the answer to these questions is yes. Scientists have been able to map some of the proposed types of memory to specific areas of the brain. Shown below are regions of nerve cells thought to be associated with the short- and long-term memory processes we discussed.

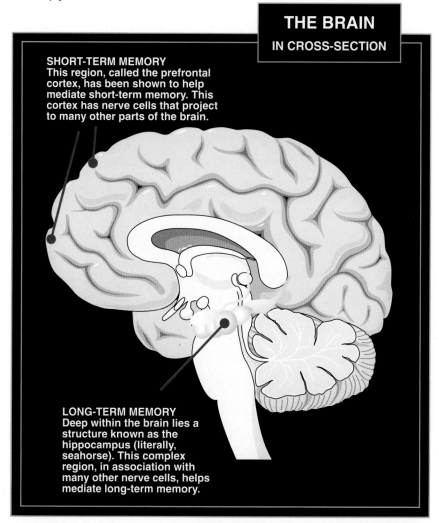

THE BRAIN
IN CROSS-SECTION

SHORT-TERM MEMORY
This region, called the prefrontal cortex, has been shown to help mediate short-term memory. This cortex has nerve cells that project to many other parts of the brain.

LONG-TERM MEMORY
Deep within the brain lies a structure known as the hippocampus (literally, seahorse). This complex region, in association with many other nerve cells, helps mediate long-term memory.

This brief map is certainly not the whole picture regarding human memory. The brain is so complex and so interconnected that we have only the roughest outline of the areas where memory takes place, even after many years of research. There is hope that we may someday obtain a more finely detailed picture of how our brains mediate memory, however. And part of this understanding may come from studying a tragic experiment of nature, the human behavior that comes from victims of stroke. How strokes may help us is described on the next page.

We have only the roughest outline of the areas where memory takes place.

Strokes are caused by leakages of blood vessels within the brain or by clots sent to, or forming within, those vessels. Brain damage occurs. Such localized destruction can result in a loss of specific brain function or changes in behavior that can sometimes be extraordinary.

WHAT WE'VE LEARNED FROM STROKES

By correlating the damaged area of the brain with the change in function or behavior, scientists obtain clues as to which regions govern which functions. This includes, among other things, the fine structure of human memory. Here are three examples:

FACES

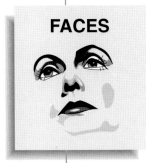

A middle-aged mother of three woke up one morning and, to her horror, could not recognize her husband or her children. Terrified, she was taken to a hospital where she was diagnosed with a stroke. The area of the brain that was damaged destroyed her ability to recognize *any* face, not just her family's (such a condition is called *prosopagnosia*). This demonstrates that an area of the brain holds the key to facial recognition. This area was damaged by the stroke.

ANIMALS

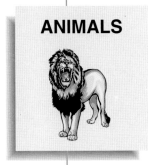

An older man suffered a stroke that left him unable to recognize pictures of animals. But only the pictures. If he were presented with the written name of the animal, he could identify the creature accurately. He could even draw the animal he just described. Incredibly, when his own drawing was shown to him and he was asked to identify the creature, he could not. This demonstrated that graphical memories of objects like animals, and the texts that describe them, are stored separately. The stroke, at some level, may have broken the connection between these areas.

LANGUAGE

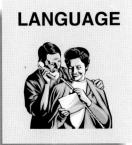

Language deficits are common in stroke victims. Some have trouble using and understanding nouns, for example. Others can understand nouns just fine, but have trouble with verbs. Some stroke victims can't produce language, though they can understand it perfectly. Others speak just fine, but might as well be deaf; they have lost the ability to understand what they hear. How this relates structurally is only just beginning to become clear. Regardless, the data point out that at some level, specific verbal functions can be separated and then stored in separate areas.

THE IMPORTANCE OF COMPARTMENTS

These deficits provide tantalizing glimpses into the fine structure of human memory. As you probably noticed, these stroke-induced behaviors are reminiscent of the behaviors of people with Alzheimer's disease. Though it is impossible to make specific correlations, both diseases illustrate the extreme compartmentalization of the brain. And the effect that one crippled compartment can have on an otherwise perfectly functioning organ. The existence of regional specialization is one of the most important facts to remember in our attempt to make sense of the sometimes baffling behavior of Alzheimer's patients.

CHAPTER
FOUR

*Nerve cells and
the genetic code*

What a nerve cell looks like

Nerve cells come in many shapes and sizes. Regardless of their form, these important cells have many structures in common.

10/13/89

The fault thing. Am I ever going to get over the fault thing? Today had some very embarrassing moments. It all had to do with Dr. Kramer coming over early, and completely unannounced, I might add. I was scolding Daddy for messing up the closet in his room. Daddy responded with his usual withdrawal, but as I was talking to him (Kramer said later I was shouting), I heard the doorbell ring. And it was Kramer. He asked if he could see Daddy, which he did for about 15 minutes. Then he asked if he could talk to me tomorrow. His tone of voice made me scared, but I said he could come over again. I think he overheard me lecturing Daddy and I think he's going to chew me out.

It is common for caregivers like Beth to become frustrated with the people in their care. As we have discussed, a disease of the brain can lead to behaviors that appear deliberate in the person who is sick. One of the reasons we are addressing the inner workings of Alzheimer's is to provide a clearer picture of just how much a *physical* disease AD is, and to communicate that "fault" is not an issue.

If the last chapter was devoted to larger structures such as memory systems and regions of the brain, this chapter is devoted to much smaller structures, such as nerve cells and the molecules that inhabit them. We begin by examining the anatomy of a typical nerve cell.

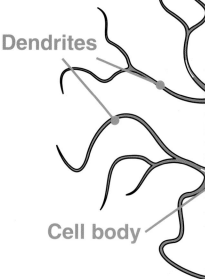

Dendrites

Cell body

NERVE CELL ARCHITECTURE

As you know, the brain is made of nerve cells, usually called neurons. The brain contains over 100 billion individual neurons, which means there are as many nerve cells in one human head as there are stars in the entire Milky Way galaxy!

Shown here is the structure of a typical, generalized neuron. In order to understand how Alzheimer's works, we will need to understand the overall construction of human nerve cells. This structure can be divided into three regions.

1

The overall structure of a neuron makes it look something like a spider web on a stick. The center of the web-like structure is called the *cell body*. This area houses the command center for the entire cell, including all the genetic information.

The cell body also possesses finger-like projections that extend into the outer environs, giving the nerve its web-like appearance. Those projections are called *dendrites*, from the Greek word *dendros*, which means tree. Nerve cells use these dendrites to communicate information to neighboring neurons.

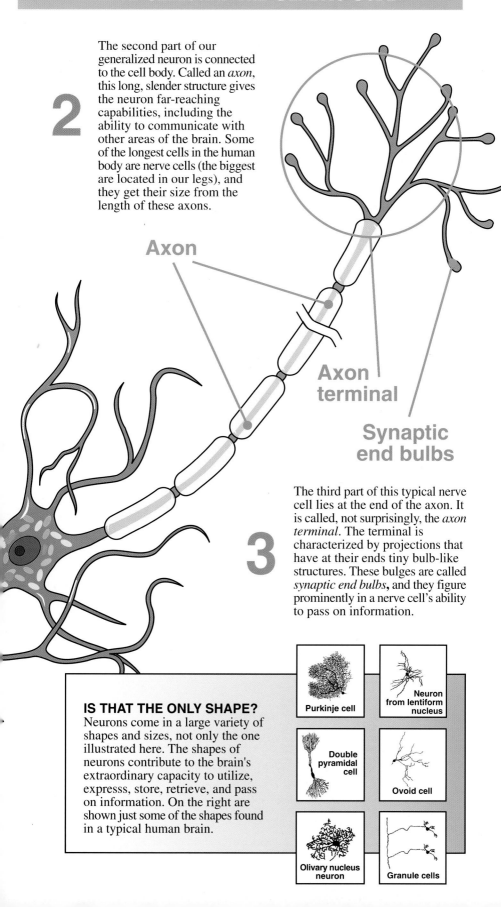

2 The second part of our generalized neuron is connected to the cell body. Called an *axon*, this long, slender structure gives the neuron far-reaching capabilities, including the ability to communicate with other areas of the brain. Some of the longest cells in the human body are nerve cells (the biggest are located in our legs), and they get their size from the length of these axons.

Axon

Axon terminal

Synaptic end bulbs

3 The third part of this typical nerve cell lies at the end of the axon. It is called, not surprisingly, the *axon terminal*. The terminal is characterized by projections that have at their ends tiny bulb-like structures. These bulges are called *synaptic end bulbs,* and they figure prominently in a nerve cell's ability to pass on information.

IS THAT THE ONLY SHAPE?
Neurons come in a large variety of shapes and sizes, not only the one illustrated here. The shapes of neurons contribute to the brain's extraordinary capacity to utilize, expresss, store, retrieve, and pass on information. On the right are shown just some of the shapes found in a typical human brain.

Purkinje cell

Neuron from lentiform nucleus

Double pyramidal cell

Ovoid cell

Olivary nucleus neuron

Granule cells

Command and control

All neurons have a spherical structure inside their cell bodies. Called a nucleus, this structure commands and controls most functions of a nerve cell.

10/14/89

I guess I was a bit more nervous than I needed to be. Kramer came over this evening. My heart skipped a beat or two when I heard him ring the doorbell. He really *did* want to talk to me about the yelling incident he heard yesterday, but he did not come to chew me out. Instead, he took out a bunch of paper clippings he had been saving. They had to do with Alzheimer's disease, and all of them concerned the latest breakthroughs in research. He told me that this might help me see Daddy's behavior as a disease. Then he told me that yelling would do no good. When Kramer left, I started going through the clippings. He underlined the first one, which had to do with describing what nerve cells looked like.

THE INSIDE OF A NEURON

When somebody with as little science background as Beth encounters the bewildering world of cellular biology, the first reaction may be to change the subject. As Beth began leafing through Kramer's news clippings, however, she began to see that the organization of a typical nerve cell is actually quite simple. For example, one of the most important structures in a neuron is also one of the easiest to see— the round ball in the cell body called a *nucleus*. The internal structure of a neuron, complete with a description of the contents of the nucleus, is shown on this page.

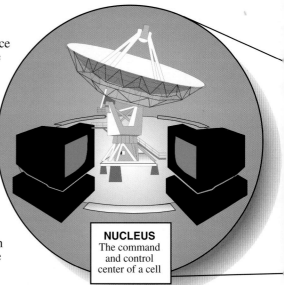

NUCLEUS
The command and control center of a cell

INSIDE THE NUCLEUS

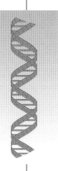

The nucleus of a neuron does not use computers and radar dishes to perform its central functions, of course. Rather, the nucleus houses most of the genetic information a cell possesses. It is this genetic information that is ultimately responsible for most of the controlling functions. The information is parcelled out into volumes, the same way an encyclopedia may be organized into various books. We call these "volumes" *chromosomes*. And chromosomes are not made out of paper, but out of a very famous molecule called *DNA*. Shown on the left is what DNA looks like, the legendary double helix.

WHAT'S OUTSIDE THE NUCLEUS

The contents of the nucleus are physically separated from the inside of the neuron by a fatty membrane. This interior, which is mostly saltwater, is called the *cytoplasm* (or sometimes, the *cytosol*).

Cytoplasm

Nucleus

DNA within the nucleus

Neurons are well-connected

Neurons, complete with their nuclei and cytoplasm, are associated in complex networks. These networks connect various regions of the brain, allowing communication.

10/16/89

I looked at more of Kramer's clippings this evening. Some of them make great night reading because they are so dull—they kind of remind me of college. His method seems to be working, though. I am already looking at Daddy in a different way when he starts to get weird. He was doing his ritualistic destruction of his closet again. But instead of blaming Daddy and shouting at him, I just put the stuff back when he took a nap.

As this entry suggests, Beth's increasing comprehension of her father's brain chemistry was allowing her to understand his behavior from a different perspective. But comprehending how neurons function requires more than just a working knowledge of the nuclei and cytoplasm discussed on the previous page. Something that helped Beth tremendously was learning that individual neurons communicate with each other incessantly, are connected in very complicated ways, and can create bizarre behavior when the communication is disrupted. How neurons connect to each other to form these communication pathways is discussed below.

how neurons communicate ...

> Neurons communicate with each other the same way computers do: they use electricity.

Neurons talk to each other like teenagers on a telephone. But they perform the task the same way computers do, by using electricity. If you stubbed your toe, for example, neurons would become electrically activated, passing the information about the injury from your foot all the way to your brain. Such information travels along the neurons as brief electrical pulses, called *action potentials*.

Communication not only exists between body parts, but also between areas within our brain. In many cases, neurons are grouped to form networks, just like wires can be grouped to form circuits. Various nerve cells have to be specifically associated with other nerve cells to carry out tasks within the brain. Most relevant to Alzheimer's, those tasks may not be executed if neurons within the circuit are destroyed.

INTRICACIES IN ONE CELL

Though the networks like the one below can be quite complex, the connections between individual nerve cells can be just as intricate. Pictured on the left is a neuron known as a Purkinje cell. This nerve cell is located deep within the cerebellum, the brain region responsible for coordinating physical movement. Possessing a virtual wilderness of connecting parts, a single Purkinje fiber may associate with as many as 100,000 other neurons!

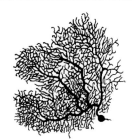

A single Purkinje cell, a neuron located deep within the cerebellum.

EXAMPLE OF A NETWORK

Neurons form multi-cellular networks within the brain. Shown here is one such network, called the dopaminergic pathway. This pathway is important in mediating both mood and movement.

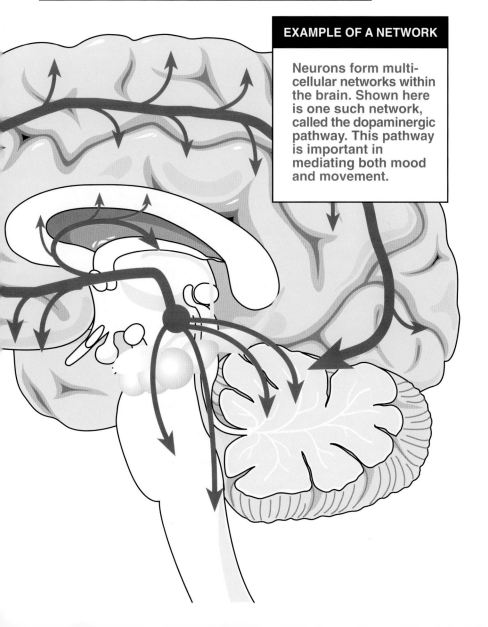

The space between neurons

Though adjacent neurons can transfer information to each other, they are not physically connected. A gap called a synapse exists between neighboring neurons.

10/18/89

Kramer came over last night again. This time he asked me how my "lessons" were going. I was kind of in a sullen mood because I had yelled at Daddy again earlier this morning. I thanked him for his newspaper clippings, and told him that they had made a difference. I said that I now stare at Daddy's head and wonder what Daddy's nerve connections are doing. It wasn't a total lie, but Kramer seemed to see through it. He laughed and handed me a magazine article about genes and Alzheimer's. I told him I would read it, which is probably true. But I hope he doesn't come over for awhile.

We have been discussing the fact that neurons form networks within the brain, allowing various regions to communicate. The implication, which Beth addressed when she told Kramer about staring at Daddy's head, is that the neurons are somehow spliced together. Nerve cells *are* connected to each other, though exactly how might surprise you. Those connections and how they work are the subject of the next couple of pages. We begin with a space researchers call a *synapse*.

THE CONNECTIONS AREN'T PHYSICAL

Though individual neurons form complex networks with adjacent nerve cells, there is *no* physical connection between the cells. Instead, a space exists between one neuron and its immediate neighbor. This space is termed a synapse, which comes from a Latin word meaning "connection."

Because of the existence of synapses, electrical impulses cannot jump from one nerve cell to the next. Instead, a stimulated nerve cell has to find a way to transfer information across the gap so that its neighbor will understand what is being communicated. If the gap is successfully crossed, the neighbor will react and the signal will be transferred. If the gap is not successfully crossed, the information will not be transferred (we will talk about how this is done later). Shown on the right is a simple illustration of a synapse between two nerve cells.

Though the illustration shows only a single connection, most neurons possess many synapses between themselves and their neighbors (like those Purkinje cells on the previous page). Why so many connections? The answer has to do with the significance a single synapse has on a neuron. When considered individually, synapses usually produce only a small effect on a neighboring nerve cell. Most neurons, however, are capable of reading literally hundreds of inputs from multiple synapses, and a given cell may *need* multiple inputs before it will react. Thus, it may be better to think of individual nerve cells like smart computers, rather than as dumb wires, in transferring information from one point to the next. They have the ability to integrate and make decisions based upon patterns received from an enormous number of inputs.

A synapse is the space that exists between neurons

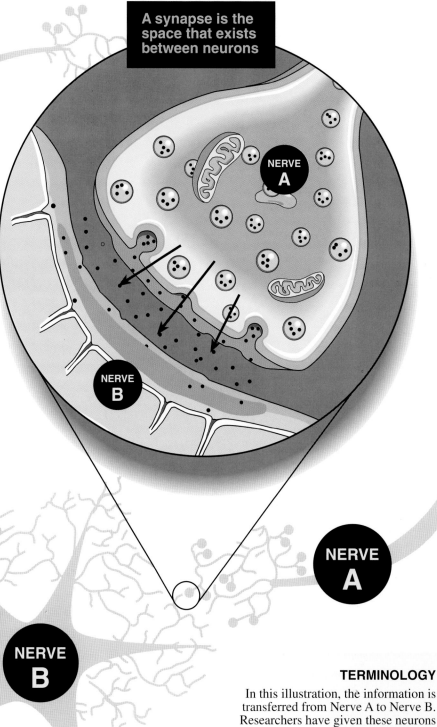

NERVE A

NERVE B

NERVE A

NERVE B

TERMINOLOGY

In this illustration, the information is transferred from Nerve A to Nerve B. Researchers have given these neurons special names because of the flow of information. Nerve A is called the *presynaptic neuron* because it is transferring information to the synapse. Nerve B is called the *postsynaptic neuron* because it is receiving the information from the synapse.

Crossing the neural gap

How does information get across the synapse? Neurons use chemicals called neurotransmitters to transfer information from one nerve cell to the next.

On the previous page, we discussed the gaps that exist between communicating neurons. If information is to be transferred, the natural question is: How do they get across the gap?

Fortunately, a great deal is known about how information crosses the space between nerve cells. Neurons transfer information to each other by using small, mobile chemicals. These chemicals, termed *neurotransmitters,* come in a variety of types. Neurotransmitters are stored in bags called *vesicles* (see below). These chemical-filled bags stay inside the nerve cell until they are needed.

Facing the cell with the neurotransmitters, the neurons on the other side of the synapse possess a class of molecules known as *receptors.* They are tethered to the cell's surface edge, projecting outward into the synapse. Receptors have two jobs: a) they bind to neurotransmitters and b) tell the cell to which they are anchored that a neurotransmitter has been received.

AN EXAMPLE OF HOW THEY WORK

Pictured below are two neurons, A and B. The goal is to transfer information from Neuron A to Neuron B by crossing the synaptic gap. The neurotransmitters, colored as red spheres, are stored in their vesicles in Neuron A. Neuron B has receptors on its surface (pictured in yellow) that can bind to the A's neurotransmitters.

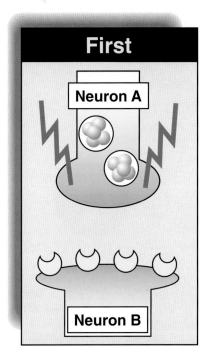

First

Neuron A

Neuron B

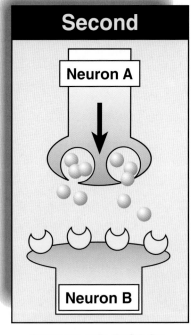

Second

Neuron A

Neuron B

STEP #1: NEURON "A" RECEIVES A SIGNAL
The process begins when Neuron A becomes electrically stimulated. This stimulation can occur for a variety of reasons, from a dancer stubbing a toe to a scholar reading a textbook. The goal is transfer the stimulation from A to B.

STEP #2: RELEASE OF NEUROTRANSMITTERS
Whatever the source of stimulation, the vesicles move to the outer edge of the neuron as a result. They quickly release their contents of neurotransmitters into the gap between Neurons A and B.

HOW FAST DOES IT GO?

As seen below, nerve cells use a combination of electricity and chemistry to communicate with each other. How quickly does information get transferred? The answer, surprisingly, is that nerve cells are quite slow. The reason is that neurons aren't very effective cables. The electrical signal we discussed earlier can start at one end of a nerve cell, but must frequently be regenerated to get the signal through its entire length. The maximum speed a signal can go is about 3,000 feet per second. That's one-millionth of the speed at which electricity moves through a copper wire. Because of the slowness, complex thoughts must depend on the timing of many impulses distributed over nerve cells working in parallel. Such cooperation is extremely important to performing everyday tasks. When a network of neurons loses some of its individual members, as they can with Alzheimer's, cooperation can be altered or extinguished. Loss of mental function may result.

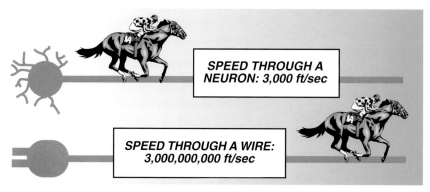

SPEED THROUGH A NEURON: 3,000 ft/sec

SPEED THROUGH A WIRE: 3,000,000,000 ft/sec

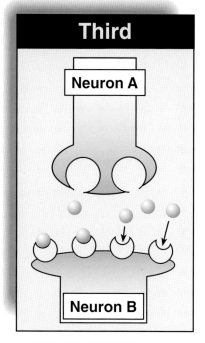

Third

Neuron A

Neuron B

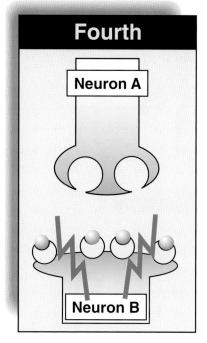

Fourth

Neuron A

Neuron B

STEP #3: BINDING TO A RECEPTOR
The newly released neurotransmitters quickly traverse the gap between the neurons. If they float close enough to the surface of Neuron B, they will bind to the receptors on the nerve cell's surface.

STEP #4: THE SIGNAL IS TRANSFERRED
The binding of neurotransmitter to receptor results in communicating information to Neuron B. It becomes electrically stimulated, just as Neuron A had before. The signal has been successfully transferred across the gap.

A brief review

A summary of what's been covered is provided below. This is done in preparation for a discussion about genes and their role in Alzheimer's disease, coming next.

10/20/89

I started reading the magazine article Kramer gave me and it has scared me to death! It said that there were genes that caused certain kinds of Alzheimer's disease! I had no idea there were actually *kinds* of Alzheimer's and I certainly didn't know that there were genes. Doesn't that mean if there are genes that they could be inherited? Like eye color? Like I could get it from Daddy? I tried calling Kramer about a hundred times, but he wasn't home. Now I don't think I'll be getting a lot of sleep tonight, and I don't think I will let him give me any more articles.

We have been talking for quite awhile about nerve cells and how they work. Left out of the discussion is an issue Beth stumbled upon when she read about Alzheimer's and specific genes. That is, why do nerve cells work the way they do? What happens when Alzheimer's appears? Are there really types of Alzheimer's, and can they be inherited?

In the next few pages, we will describe the background necessary to answer some of these questions. First, however, we will briefly review some of the concepts about neurons we just discussed. On the next page, we will begin a journey into the tiniest world in all biology, a world that holds the keys to understanding Alzheimer's disease at its most intimate level. This is the realm of the nucleus of a nerve cell and its very famous resident, the molecules of DNA.

The last few pages ...

1 We first discussed the fact that the human brain is made of closely packed cells called neurons. We found that there are several parts to a neuron, and that nerve cells come in a variety of shapes. We also learned that these sophisticated cells are highly organized, forming complex pathways in the brain.

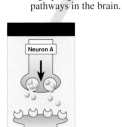

2 We next described that neurons are connected and that they use these associations to be in constant communication with each other. We learned that they share information with one another using electrical signals. Surprisingly, we found that connected neurons do not touch each other, but are separated by a gap termed a synapse.

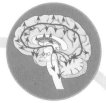

3 Our last discussion centered around how the information in a neuron crosses the gap and is transferred to a receiving neuron. We discovered that neurons use tiny chemicals called neurotransmitters. An electrically stimulated neuron will send out these chemicals. The neurotransmitters cross the gap and land on receptors waiting for them on the opposite neuron. This landing then electrically stimulates the opposite neuron and the information is passed on.

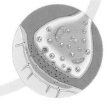

of genes, DNA and Alzheimer's disease ...

With the review of nerve cells in mind, we are ready to begin our discussion of genes and Alzheimer's. At the start of this chapter, we explained that cells can be divided into two regions: the sphere-shaped nucleus sitting in the center, and the rest of cell, called the cytoplasm (or cytosol).

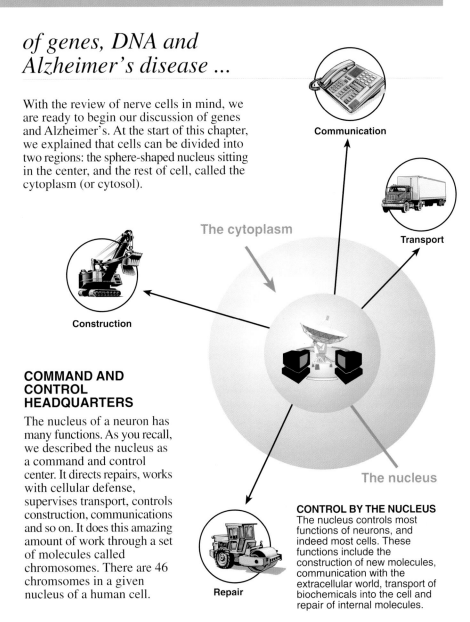

Communication

Transport

The cytoplasm

Construction

The nucleus

Repair

COMMAND AND CONTROL HEADQUARTERS

The nucleus of a neuron has many functions. As you recall, we described the nucleus as a command and control center. It directs repairs, works with cellular defense, supervises transport, controls construction, communications and so on. It does this amazing amount of work through a set of molecules called chromosomes. There are 46 chromsomes in a given nucleus of a human cell.

CONTROL BY THE NUCLEUS

The nucleus controls most functions of neurons, and indeed most cells. These functions include the construction of new molecules, communication with the extracellular world, transport of biochemicals into the cell and repair of internal molecules.

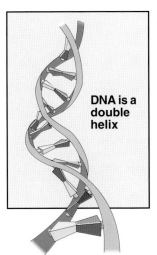

DNA is a double helix

WHAT CHROMOSOMES ARE MADE OF

As we discussed, chromosomes are composed of a molecule called *DNA* (standing for the tongue-twisting term deoxyribonucleic acid). DNA looks like a rubber ladder that has been twisted at one end. We call this structure a double helix. What does such an oddly shaped structure do that makes it the municipal governing organization of an entire neuron? The simplicity of the answer might surprise you.

The simple function of DNA

DNA resides in the nucleus of all human cells, including neurons. Despite its important job, DNA actually performs a simple function, described below.

As we discussed, chromosomes are really long strands of DNA. You might think that the heart of the command and control center might have extremely complex functions, considering the importance of the task. The nucleus *is* a complex structure, no question about it. But the DNA inside has a surprisingly simple function. Here it is:

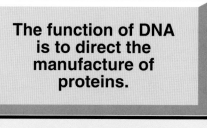

The function of DNA is to direct the manufacture of proteins.

Proteins. The same familiar molecules found in ...

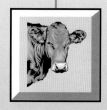

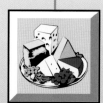

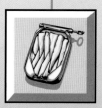

... steak ...   ... and cheese ...   ... and even sardines.

JUST PROTEINS?

At first glance, DNA's function might not sound like much, considering all there is to control in a neuron (or indeed any cell). But encoding instructions for making proteins is just what DNA does, and in so doing, the molecule controls the whole cell. To understand the importance of this simple function, let's now look at the role that proteins play in our bodies and cells.

The importance of proteins in our bodies and in our neurons

OUR BODIES

Proteins play two overall roles in our bodies. The first one is structural. Our muscles are made of protein, and the reason they have their shape and all load-bearing properties is the presence of proteins. Proteins help keep the outer skin glued to our bodies. Our hair is made of proteins. Our fingernails and toenails are too. We would not exist in our present shape without them. In fact, we would not exist at all.

Proteins also play a *functional* role in our bodies. They supervise many kinds of chemical reactions, reactions we must have in order to survive. Such proteins are often called *enzymes*, and they control functions such as digestion, breathing, circulation, reproduction, waste elimination, indeed most of the functions humans need to live.

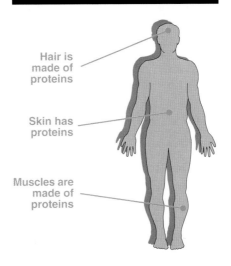

Human body

Hair is made of proteins

Skin has proteins

Muscles are made of proteins

OUR NEURONS

More to our discussion, proteins play a critical role in the functioning of nerve cells. They supervise the construction of neurotransmitters, for example, which can themselves be made of protein. Most receptors on the surface of neurons, like those which can bind to neurotransmitters, are made of proteins. Even the transmission of the electrical signal across the nerve cell occurs because of proteins. Called *ion channels*, these proteins perform this vital function by selectively allowing charges to move in and out of a given nerve, aiding the propagation of the electrical signal.

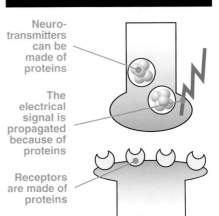

Neurons

Neuro-transmitters can be made of proteins

The electrical signal is propagated because of proteins

Receptors are made of proteins

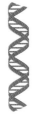

BUT HOW DOES DNA DO IT?

How can DNA, this long, twisted ladder of a molecule in the cell's nucleus, encode the information necessary to make these vital proteins? To begin with, DNA only *possesses* the information necessary to make proteins. It cannot by itself make them. Does that mean other structures have to create proteins? And if so, how does all this relate to Alzheimer's? The point of this book is to explain the disease in as close a detail as possible. That means we have to answer these questions.

Of necklaces and pretzels

What is the relationship between proteins and DNA? The answer is found by looking at their internal structures.

10/25/89

Tonight Kramer returned my phone call. I don't know whether he put my mind at ease, though. Mostly he just said that only a few cases of Alzheimer's appear to have "a strong genetic basis," whatever that means. He also said that there's a lot that nobody knows, and that you can't predict from anybody's case (like Daddy's) if a relative (like me) is going to get the disease. And then he tried to tell me about the genetic code. The surprising thing is that I actually understood him a little.

As Beth hints in the entry above, modern genetics can be understood by almost anybody. For example, we have seen that the main duty of DNA is actually quite simple: it encodes information to make proteins. We really do mean the word "code." In fact, the information on the DNA is called the genetic code, and if we could understand it, we would know a lot about our cells. Maybe even a lot about Alzheimer's. Several decades ago, this genetic code was broken, and now scientists can explain the relationship between DNA and proteins. This relationship is critically important for understanding Alzheimer's. And it *is* easy to learn. For us to discuss its function and its relevance to AD, we first need to describe the molecules.

BEADED NECKLACES

The best way to explain what DNA looks like is to envision a beaded necklace that has been cut at one end. Let's say the beads on this broken necklace come in one of four different colors. When you look at it closely, you see that the colors are arranged in a seemingly random pattern. There might be a yellow one, followed by perhaps two red ones, then maybe a blue one, perhaps another yellow, then two green ones and so on.

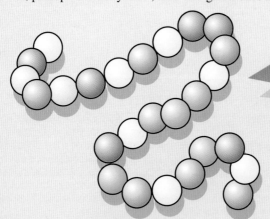

HOW DOES A BEADED NECKLACE LOOK LIKE A DNA MOLECULE?

DNA really does look a bit like a necklace that's been cut. The big difference is that DNA is not made of four different kinds of beads, but four different kinds of chemicals. We call these chemicals *nucleotides.* The nucleotides are symbolized with letters instead of colors. These letters are A, G, T, and C. Just like the necklace, when you look closely at a strand of DNA, you see letters arranged in a pattern that appears arbitrary. There might be one A, followed by two Ts, followed by a C, an A, maybe two more Gs, and so on. The difference between DNA and a necklace, however, is that this pattern is anything but random.

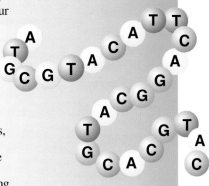

BUT ISN'T DNA A DOUBLE HELIX?

Yes. DNA is actually composed of two separate strands, not just a linear series of beads. If we continue with our jewelry metaphor, imagine one beaded necklace that has been intertwined with another beaded necklace. That's more what DNA looks like. The fact that there are two strands is where the word *double* comes from; the word *helix* refers to their being intertwined in a spiral configuration.

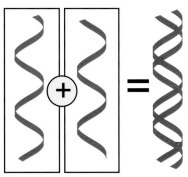

DNA is composed of two strands.

AND WHAT ABOUT PROTEINS?

The other class of molecules we have been discussing are proteins, whose manufacture, as previously explained, gives DNA its purpose. If one looks closely at proteins, it will be discovered that they look somewhat like a pretzel, with all kinds of curving twists and turns. Though convoluted, proteins are also made of component parts, just like DNA. But there are two big differences when proteins are compared to DNA: 1) Proteins are not composed of different kinds of nucleotides. Rather, proteins are composed of individual subunits called *amino acids.* This is not like the acid that exists in a common automobile battery. Amino acids are a different—and much less lethal—kind of acid. 2) There are not just four kinds of chemicals from which to choose, as with DNA. Rather, proteins can use over 20 different amino acids in their structure. But amino acids *are* reminiscent of nucleotides in that they are lined up like the beads on a necklace. Unlike DNA, proteins get folded and then refolded. This folding is so dramatic that most proteins look like a pretzel, hence our metaphor.

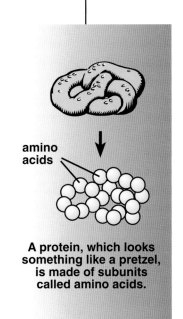

amino
acids

A protein, which looks something like a pretzel, is made of subunits called amino acids.

The relationship between necklaces and pretzels

There is a direct and functional relationship between DNA and proteins. It all has to do with the individual subunits of which these two classes of molecules are composed.

10/26/89

I called Amy and told her about my talks with Dr. Kramer. She's still kind of a science geek after all these years, and she seemed totally unconcerned about genes and Alzheimer's and Daddy. She said *she* had learned about the genetic code in 8th grade - and then she told me that *I* had too. I honestly couldn't remember, which of course made me start to worry about whether I was coming down with Alzheimer's.

THE GENETIC CODE

In the above entry, when referring to the genetic code Amy was really talking to her sister about nucleotides and amino acids. While it has long since been broken, the code was mysterious to researchers a few decades ago. In a question reminiscent of mixed metaphors like necklaces and pretzels, they asked: how could nucleotides possibly be related to amino acids? If DNA was the command and control center, would they not direct protein construction? Could nucleotides, if grouped together, somehow specify the instructions for an amino acid?

The answer to this question turned out to be yes. Eventually, it was confirmed that the relationship between amino acids and nucleotides formed the basis of the genetic code, and it all had to do with grouping. In simple terms, the code works like this: *every three nucleotides specifies one amino acid*. This code, and how it works, is summarized below.

EACH SET OF THREE NUCLEOTIDES

A T C   C G G   A C T

Amino acid 1   Amino acid 2   Amino acid 3

SPECIFIES ONE AMINO ACID

A group of three nucleotides codes for one amino acid. Discovered in the early 1960s, this association between nucleotides and amino acids is the heart of the genetic code. A protein might have 300 amino acids in it, folded over as we previously discussed. The piece of DNA encoding the protein would then be 900 nucleotides in length.

CHANGING A LETTER

What does this have to do with Alzheimer's? The answer lies in understanding the terrifying fragility of the genetic code. For example, if you change even *one* letter in the DNA, you can quite easily change the amino acid originally specified. The function of the protein that carries the new amino acid may be altered as a result. We call such changes mutations, and the resultant alterations showing up in the proteins can be quite harmful. As we'll discover, mutations in DNA may have a great deal to do with Alzheimer's disease. Shown below is how one change in the DNA can specify a new amino acid in the protein.

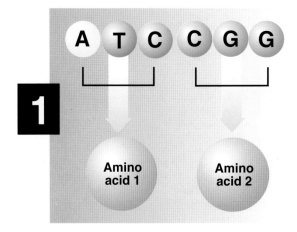

1 Here are two triplets of DNA. The first triplet (ATC) codes for amino acid 1, the other triplet (CGG), amino acid 2.

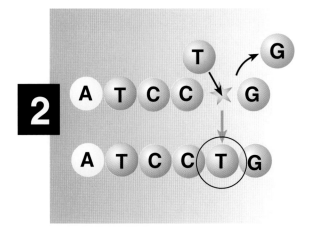

2 A change in the middle letter of the second triplet occurs. The middle "G" is removed and replaced with a "T". The sequence now reads ATCCTG, rather than ATCCGG.

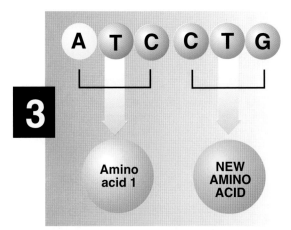

3 As a result of the switch, the second triplet no longer specifies amino acid 2. Instead, it specifies a new amino acid. The protein is now structurally (and perhaps functionally) altered. Such switches may be responsible for certain kinds of Alzheimer's.

Solving a big problem

DNA exists in a place different from that where the manufacturing sites create the proteins. How does the information from the DNA get to those sites?

Understanding the relationship between nucleotides and amino acids was a profound achievement. It opened for us an entire world of research biology, a world that eventually touched people interested in Alzheimer's research. As soon as the code was deciphered, however, scientists were confronted with a big problem.

As you know, DNA sits in the nucleus. It is incarcerated in its tiny prison, sentenced for life, with no way to get out. As this confined DNA was being characterized, another permanent jailing was discovered. This concerned the manufacturing plants that actually made the proteins, structures that could read the genetic code, find the amino acids and string them together. Termed *ribosomes*, these plants existed only outside the nucleus, just as permanently as the DNA was anchored within. So the big question was: How could a protein possibly get made if the instructions for its creation were in one place and the plant that could read the code and make the protein in another?

Nucleus

MESSAGE

← GENE

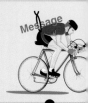
Message

This problem was eventually solved. It was discovered that cells have their own built-in copy machines and courier service. How it works is outlined in these four steps.

1 MAKING A MESSENGER

As suggested above, the nuclei of all cells have molecular copy machines inside them. These machines, a group of biochemicals, duplicate small regions of DNA, the regions containing instructions about how to make a particular protein. Scientists call these little copied messages, properly enough, *messenger RNA*, or simply mRNA.

2 LEAVING THE NUCLEUS

Here's where the courier service comes in. The nucleus possesses molecules that can shuttle the message to the outside world. Essentially, these molecules pick up the messenger RNA, escorting it out of the nucleus and into the cell's cytosol. This is how the problem of mobility is solved. The DNA does not have to leave the nucleus because it can create a portable messenger that will do the work.

3 MAKING THE PROTEIN

The next step is to get the message to the protein manufacturing plants (those ribosomes we discussed earlier). Most cells have a great number of these plants. Once the message leaves the nucleus, other escort molecules find the message and go directly to the plants. Once there, the instructions are read and the molecules at the manufacturing site go to work. They read that triplet code we talked about, find the appropriate amino acid, and then make the long chain of protein.

Cytosol

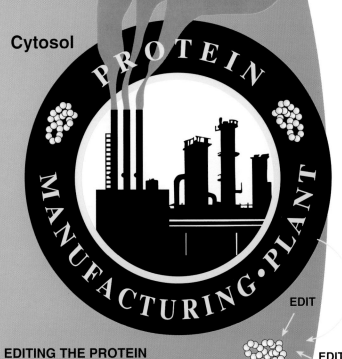

EDIT

4 EDITING THE PROTEIN

The steps outlined describe how a protein is made, even if the DNA and manufacturing sites exist in different places. But one more step usually occurs before the protein becomes useful to the cell.

EDIT

The protein coming out of the manufacturing plant is often in a "raw" form, almost as if it were the rough draft of a novel. Some kind of editing step is needed before the protein is rendered useful to the cell. Sure enough, other molecules exist outside the manufacturing plant that work like editors. Sometimes the protein has to be clipped, as if some molecular chapter were being cut from the protein. Sometimes additional molecules have to be added. Sometimes both happen. Only when this editing stage is finished, which is different for different molecules, will the protein be ready for work within the cell. As we'll see later, this editing process is very important for understanding the molecules that may be responsible for Alzheimer's disease.

Of genes and a review

We have covered a lot of material. After a brief comment about genes, we review the molecular portion of this chapter.

We have one last concept to discuss before we review the molecular part of this chapter. Dr. Kramer consistently used the word *gene* when he was talking to Beth, but he never really defined it for her. A gene is a special region of a chromosome that is made of DNA. What's so special about a gene? A gene is the region of DNA that gets copied into messenger RNA. As we'll see in the next chapter, genes play a very important role in our understanding of Alzheimer's disease. Before we get into the genes themselves, let's briefly review the material covered in the second part of this chapter.

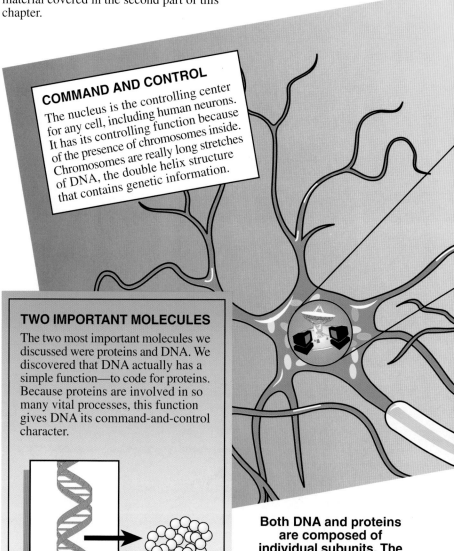

COMMAND AND CONTROL
The nucleus is the controlling center for any cell, including human neurons. It has its controlling function because of the presence of chromosomes inside. Chromosomes are really long stretches of DNA, the double helix structure that contains genetic information.

TWO IMPORTANT MOLECULES
The two most important molecules we discussed were proteins and DNA. We discovered that DNA actually has a simple function—to code for proteins. Because proteins are involved in so many vital processes, this function gives DNA its command-and-control character.

DNA encodes the information necessary to make proteins.

Both DNA and proteins are composed of individual subunits. The subunits in a DNA molecule are called nucleotides. The subunits in a protein molecule are called amino acids.

The genetic code is a description of how groups of nucleotides specify individual amino acids.

The relationship between nucleotides and amino acids is direct. The genetic code is read in groups of three nucleotides. Every triplet specifies an individual amino acid on a protein. If a protein is composed of 300 amino acids, that means the DNA had to use 900 nucleotides to properly code for it.

Mistakes can occur in the genetic code. These errors are termed mutations. We examined one such mistake, the substitution of one nucleotide for another. When this occurs, a different amino acid may be specified than exists in the normal protein. This can be disastrous. The genetic code is so delicate that even a single nucleotide change in one chromosome (producing the abnormal protein) can hurt an entire organism. Indeed, certain kinds of Alzheimer's disease may be the fault of mutations in the DNA of the patient. That is why we study this biology here.

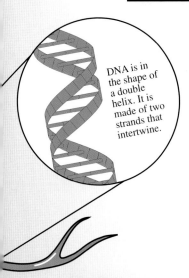

DNA is in the shape of a double helix. It is made of two strands that intertwine.

TWO IMPORTANT MOLECULES

We last talked about how cells solve the following problem: the DNA is in the nucleus and the protein manufacturing site (the ribosome) is in the cytosol. How this problem is solved involves the creation of a messenger. The entire process is summarized below.

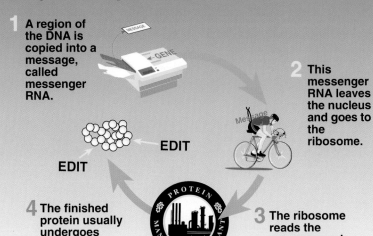

1 A region of the DNA is copied into a message, called messenger RNA.

2 This messenger RNA leaves the nucleus and goes to the ribosome.

3 The ribosome reads the message and creates a protein based on what the message encodes.

4 The finished protein usually undergoes some kind of editing after it leaves the ribosome.

EDIT

EDIT

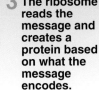

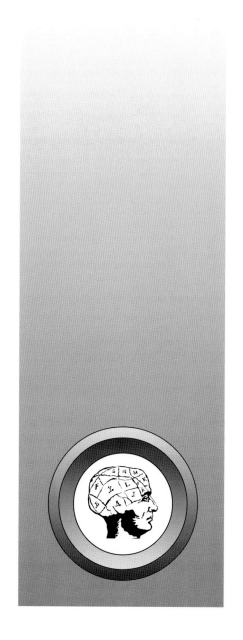

CHAPTER
FIVE

*Why Alzheimer's
destroys the brain*

Introduction to the chapter

We are now ready to talk discuss in detail the biology of Alzheimer's.

2/4/90

Daddy was yelling at the top of his lungs. "Where are my books?," was all he could say, over and over and over again! I tried to shut myself off in my room, but he kept shouting louder and louder. Finally, I went downstairs to the den. There was Daddy, cross-legged on the floor, pointing at an empty space in his book closet. Sure enough, there were some books missing. When he saw me come into the room he began pointing at his head and repeating his tirade. "Where are my books?!" This went on for another 10 minutes before he stormed out of the den. He pushed me out of the way as he left, giving me a bruise on my arm.

Behaviors like Daddy's shouting may be understood in terms of molecules, cells, and the brain operations that coordinate them. With that knowledge in mind, we are ready to tackle a most important question: Why does Alzheimer's destroy a person's mental function? Indeed, what are the mechanisms behind the brain's sad deterioration? Does understanding how the disease works give us hints as to how we might treat it?

How we will address such vital questions is shown in the road map on the next page. We have already covered a fair amount of science in an attempt to make sense of Alzheimer's. But to understand AD at its core, we will need to cover a few more biological concepts. Let's briefly review a few facts from the previous chapters about brains and molecules before we get started on our explanation of AD. These facts are summarized below.

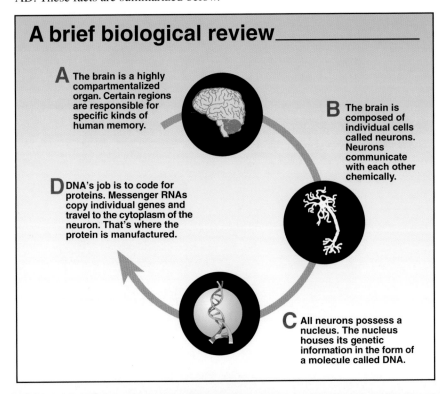

A brief biological review_____

A The brain is a highly compartmentalized organ. Certain regions are responsible for specific kinds of human memory.

B The brain is composed of individual cells called neurons. Neurons communicate with each other chemically.

C All neurons possess a nucleus. The nucleus houses its genetic information in the form of a molecule called DNA.

D DNA's job is to code for proteins. Messenger RNAs copy individual genes and travel to the cytoplasm of the neuron. That's where the protein is manufactured.

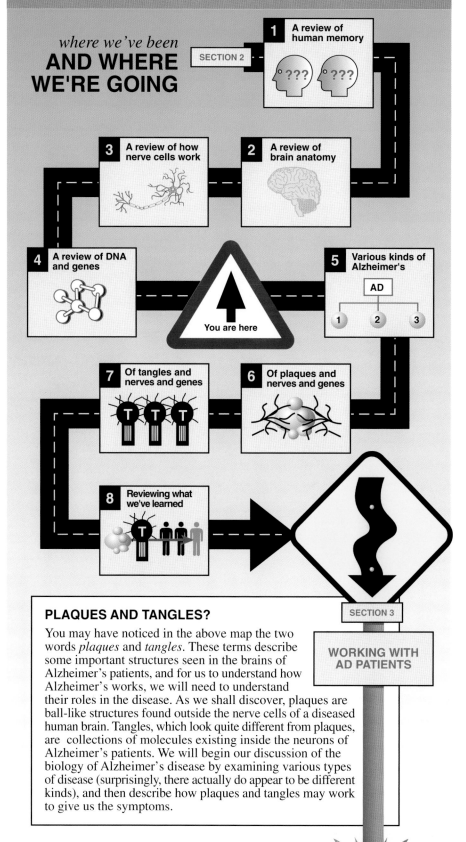

where we've been
AND WHERE WE'RE GOING

SECTION 2

1 A review of human memory

3 A review of how nerve cells work

2 A review of brain anatomy

4 A review of DNA and genes

You are here

5 Various kinds of Alzheimer's

AD

1 2 3

7 Of tangles and nerves and genes

6 Of plaques and nerves and genes

8 Reviewing what we've learned

SECTION 3

WORKING WITH AD PATIENTS

PLAQUES AND TANGLES?

You may have noticed in the above map the two words *plaques* and *tangles*. These terms describe some important structures seen in the brains of Alzheimer's patients, and for us to understand how Alzheimer's works, we will need to understand their roles in the disease. As we shall discover, plaques are ball-like structures found outside the nerve cells of a diseased human brain. Tangles, which look quite different from plaques, are collections of molecules existing inside the neurons of Alzheimer's patients. We will begin our discussion of the biology of Alzheimer's disease by examining various types of disease (surprisingly, there actually do appear to be different kinds), and then describe how plaques and tangles may work to give us the symptoms.

Types of Alzheimer's disease

AD can be classified into various types of disorders. These classifications can be based on inheritability as well as age of onset.

You might be surprised to know that there is more than one type of Alzheimer's. Thus, it may be more appropriate to think of Alzheimer's "diseases" when thinking about AD. There are a number of ways to categorize the various forms of Alzheimer's, some of which are shown here.

SPORADIC VERSUS FAMILIAL

The most general way to classify AD is to ask: Does it or doesn't it run in your family? The type of Alzheimer's disease that does not run in families is termed *sporadic Alzheimer's*. That simply means the disease arose spontaneously in the afflicted person rather than being inherited from a family member. The type of Alzheimer's that *does* show a strong genetic component is called *familial Alzheimer's disease*, or simply FAD. As the name suggests, this type of Alzheimer's disease can be inherited from a family member. FAD represents very few of the total number of Alzheimer's cases reported in this country, as shown on the chart below.

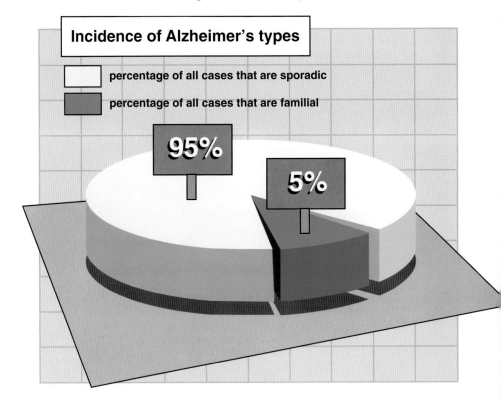

Incidence of Alzheimer's types

☐ percentage of all cases that are sporadic

■ percentage of all cases that are familial

95%

5%

HOW DO YOU KNOW IF FAD IS PRESENT?

A genetic basis for a disease always raises a terrifying question: "If a family member gets the disease, what is the chance that I will get it too?" Such concern is certainly understandable. Current research indicates that people who have an affected parent or sibling have a greater risk of developing the disease than those who don't. But that is about all you can say. A family history of AD doesn't mean that the familial type of the disease will be present in every family member. Separating out the effects of environment, viruses, head trauma, vascular disorders, etc., from the effects of any "Alzheimer's genes" is very difficult to do. With current technology, we are only just beginning to understand how various inputs can contribute to the disease. Most clinicians suspect that FAD is present only when certain criteria are met.

THE CHECKLIST

Here are some criteria doctors use to assess whether FAD exists in a given family:

Y   **N**

☑ ☐   • AD, or some other form of progressive dementia in otherwise healthy people, can be traced over several generations within a single family.

☑ ☐   • The family members shown to have had the disease also show a similar age of onset of symptoms and a similar duration of the disease.

WHICH TYPE DO WE KNOW THE MOST ABOUT?

Perhaps surprisingly, we know next to nothing about the sporadic form of Alzheimer's disease. This means the research community does not understand the origins of 95% of the cases occurring in this country. Scientists have had much greater success in understanding the mechanisms of the familial type. There is reason to believe, fortunately, that research on the inherited forms will give us hints as to the mechanisms behind the other forms. The rest of this chapter primarily will be devoted to understanding the genes behind familial Alzheimer's and how these genes contribute to the symptoms Alzheimer's patients experience.

EVEN WITHIN THE FAD CLASS THERE ARE CATEGORIES

As time goes by, it has become increasingly clear that various kinds of inherited Alzheimer's exist. As far back as 1907, Alois Alzheimer found that the disease struck people in a wide variety of ages. Now it is known that one form of FAD can afflict people in their 40s, while another kind strikes at a much later age. To distinguish between these two types, scientists call the AD that besets younger people "early-onset" and those striking older people "late-onset." How these types are distinguished from each other is shown below.

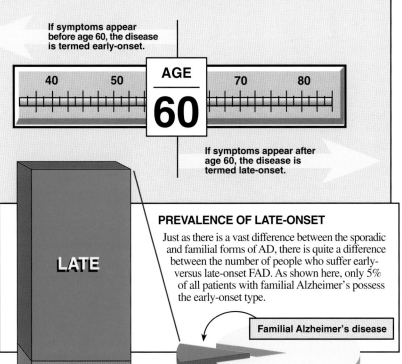

If symptoms appear before age 60, the disease is termed early-onset.

AGE
60

40   50   70   80

If symptoms appear after age 60, the disease is termed late-onset.

LATE

EARLY

PREVALENCE OF LATE-ONSET

Just as there is a vast difference between the sporadic and familial forms of AD, there is quite a difference between the number of people who suffer early- versus late-onset FAD. As shown here, only 5% of all patients with familial Alzheimer's possess the early-onset type.

Familial Alzheimer's disease

Inside an Alzheimer's brain

The brains of Alzheimer's patients look very different from the brains of unaffected individuals. They have structures known as plaques and tangles.

2/6/90

Daddy seemed to have forgotten about his missing books and magazines until yesterday. Then he started yelling again, shouting about them being stolen and pointing to his head like before. This time he also called out Bill's name and accused my brother of stealing them. Daddy became increasingly upset with each shout, so I called Bill to see if he knew anything. There was this woman's voice giggling in the background of his answering-machine message tape (new girlfriend, maybe? something I should know about?), but he hadn't returned my call as of this evening. Afterwards I went downstairs and looked in the library. Sure enough, there were more empty spaces where it looked like books should be.

When the patient, like Beth's father, is alive and functional, Alzheimer's is difficult to diagnose. To determine AD definitively, brain tissue must be examined, which usually means performing an autopsy. Dr. Alois Alzheimer was the first person to notice that the brains of people suffering from certain dementias looked abnormal at autopsy. He described what are now the two classic lesions of Alzheimer's disease, shown on the right.

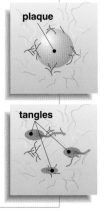

plaque

tangles

PLAQUES
Dr. Alzheimer noticed circular structures surrounded by abnormal looking nerve cells. He called these structures senile plaques.

TANGLES
He also noticed knotted thread-like structures scattered throughout the brain. He called these structures neurofibrillary tangles.

WHERE DO PLAQUES FORM?

Dr. Alzheimer noticed that the senile plaques he identified were found in specific regions of the brain. Further research has confirmed his original findings many times over. AD-related plaques are found in areas like the hippocampus, for example. This area is deeply involved in memory and learning; it makes sense that this region might be affected by the disease process. Other areas where plaques are commonly found are shown below.

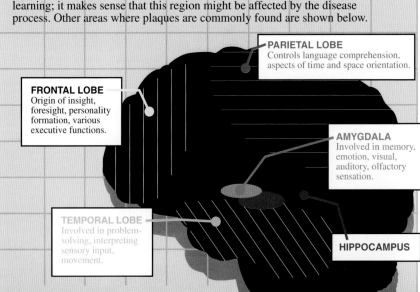

PARIETAL LOBE
Controls language comprehension, aspects of time and space orientation.

FRONTAL LOBE
Origin of insight, foresight, personality formation, various executive functions.

AMYGDALA
Involved in memory, emotion, visual, auditory, olfactory sensation.

TEMPORAL LOBE
Involved in problem-solving, interpreting sensory input, movement.

HIPPOCAMPUS

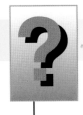

What do plaques look like?

The plaques first described by Dr. Alzheimer have two constituents. These components are shown below.

1) All plaques possess round, spherically shaped structures. These structures lie outside nerve cells and are embedded in the brain the way pieces of fruit might be embedded in gelatin. They come in a variety of sizes, ranging from very small spheres to giant, globelike structures.

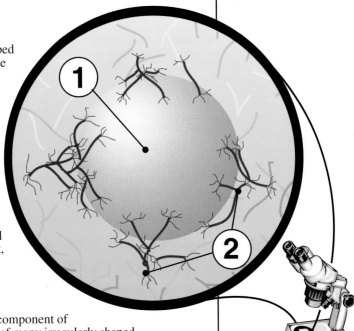

2) The second component of plaque consists of many irregularly shaped neural structures surrounding the sphere. These appear to be patches of degenerating axon terminals and dendrite branches of local neurons. A plaque is thus composed of a central globe-shaped object surrounded by what appear to be dying nerve cells.

ARE THERE ALWAYS PLAQUES?

The frustrating answer to that question (one that has been historically controversial) is no. Senile plaques can actually be found in the brains of people who underwent the normal aging process and *never* suffered from Alzheimer's. Occasionally one even finds patients who actually died of Alzheimer's disease, but showed relatively little plaque formation. How do we make sense of this data? As we shall see, the *tangles* Dr. Alzheimer discovered play a large role, maybe a determining role, in the disease many patients experience. It thus appears that plaques are not the only reason people get the symptoms of Alzheimer's (though some data suggest that a correlation between number of plaques and mental impairment exists). What the contradictory findings also show is that Alzheimer's disease is quite complex, and fully explaining why it occurs is a difficult scientific challenge.

A typical neuron looks like this

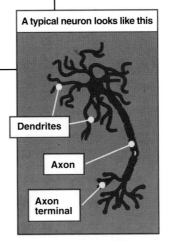

Dendrites

Axon

Axon terminal

OF WHAT ARE PLAQUES COMPOSED?

As you might expect, as soon as researchers found the plaques, they started asking questions like "What are those round spheres made of?" and "Why do surrounding nerve cells appear to be destroyed in their vicinity?" Fortunately, these questions have answers to them, answers we will discuss on the next page.

What is inside the plaques?

The sphere-shaped object found in the plaques is made of several substances. The chief constituent is a protein called beta-amyloid.

The mystery is solved! We don't have a thief in the house taking Daddy's stuff! Well, at least not an unfamiliar thief. Bill returned my phone call yesterday and fessed up to taking Daddy's books and magazines. I chewed him out royally and then asked him about the woman's voice on the phone. I guess Rachel is his new girlfriend, and she also happens to be a nurse. Bill took the book on neurology and some articles related to Alzheimer's from Daddy's bookshelf at her urging. She said she'd help him understand the disease. I calmed down pretty quickly, and after awhile even asked when the "classes" started. Now I understand why Daddy was pointing to his head when he looked at the bookshelf.

It was the winter of 1990 when Beth wrote the entry on the left in her journal. Back then, there were only hints about the biological mechanisms that caused Alzheimer's disease. Fortunately, our understanding of the disease has increased a great deal since Beth wrote those words.

For example, the contents of the round object within the plaques have been well characterized. Though complex, it has been found that one dominating molecule exists within the sphere. It is a protein called beta-amyloid 42, usually shortened to Aβ42 by scientists. What does Aβ42 have to do with Alzheimer's?

To answer that question, scientists first had to find out where Aβ42 came from. They discovered that the little protein was originally part of another, much larger molecule. To understand what they found, and how it relates to AD, we will need to discuss an important biological mechanism. This will be done in two parts: first we will quickly review what happens to proteins after they are made, and secondly, I will use an analogy. The analogy is an illustration taken from the garment industry, talking about someone Beth's father used to go to frequently: his tailor. Then we will return to the world of Alzheimer's.

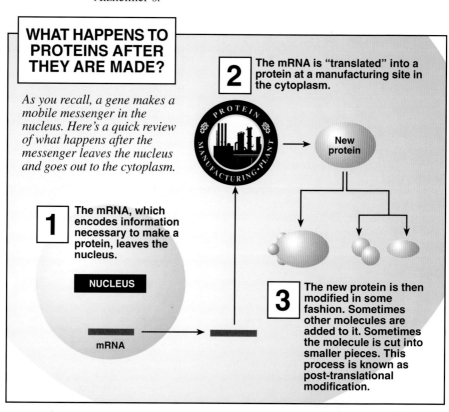

WHAT HAPPENS TO PROTEINS AFTER THEY ARE MADE?

As you recall, a gene makes a mobile messenger in the nucleus. Here's a quick review of what happens after the messenger leaves the nucleus and goes out to the cytoplasm.

1 The mRNA, which encodes information necessary to make a protein, leaves the nucleus.

NUCLEUS

mRNA

2 The mRNA is "translated" into a protein at a manufacturing site in the cytoplasm.

PROTEIN MANUFACTURING PLANT

New protein

3 The new protein is then modified in some fashion. Sometimes other molecules are added to it. Sometimes the molecule is cut into smaller pieces. This process is known as post-translational modification.

OF TAILORS AND ALZHEIMER'S

Nothing could seem further from the medical researcher's world of proteins than the tailor's world of suit manufacturing. Such a collision of environments was not lost on Beth's father. In the good doctor's healthier days, he would visit his tailor every six months or so. The tailor would patiently take Daddy's measurements and in a couple of weeks, Beth's father would have a new suit. At some stage of the manufacturing process, the tailor would have to go to a large piece of fabric. He would draw on the fabric and begin cutting out the right shapes in order to create the garment. The shapes would not be arbitrary, of course, but would have specific functions for the suit. It is obvious that without the fabric, no suit would be made. It is also obvious that if the pieces were not cut out correctly, the suit might not fit Daddy. It might never even be finished.

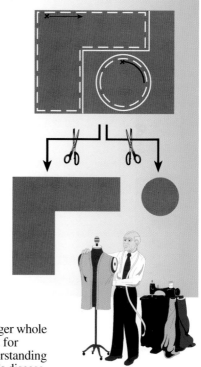

This idea of cutting distinct pieces from a larger whole for a specific function is important not just for tailoring: it is equally important for our understanding of plaques, the Aβ42 protein, and Alzheimer's disease. How they relate is described below.

BACK TO THE NEURONS

The question everybody was asking after they discovered the Aβ42 protein was this: "Where did it come from?" Scientists discovered that Aβ42 was made by nerve cells. It was actually cut from a larger protein in those cells, the same way the tailor might cut smaller pieces from a large section of fabric. This cutting is absolutely normal; it is an example of that post-translational modification we discussed on the previous page.

This larger protein has a name. It is called APP, short for *amyloid precursor protein*. In healthy individuals, APP is processed in such fashion that several smaller proteins are cleaved from the original. Some of these smaller proteins are escorted out of the cell. As is shown on the right, there are two types of proteins that leave, called Aβ40 and Aβ42. There usually is much more Aβ40 than Aβ42.

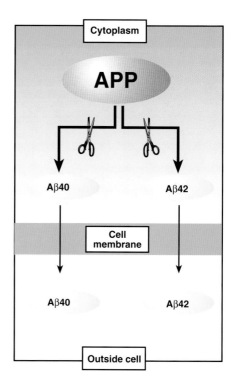

This mechanism has a great deal to do with the presence of plaques in the human brain. The reason has to do with the behavior of Aβ40 and Aβ42 once they leave the nerve cell.

Of Alzheimer's, plaques, and dying neurons

The plaques described on the previous page can be deadly to nerve cells in the brain. This toxicity may play a critical role in the symptoms of Alzheimer's disease.

From the last page we learned that the large APP molecule can be cleaved into smaller proteins. We also learned that these smaller proteins, termed $A\beta40$ and $A\beta42$, can escape the neuron. As previously mentioned, it is important to remember that healthy cells make both kinds of smaller proteins. But in normal adults, a lot more $A\beta40$ is produced than $A\beta42$ (in fact, $A\beta42$ is considered to be just a minor by-product). With this information in mind, we are ready to discuss the role of these proteins in Alzheimer's disease. Here are three important facts:

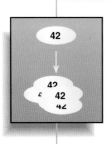

FACT #1: THE DIFFERENCE IS STICKINESS

$A\beta40$ has properties very different from those of its cousin $A\beta42$. One of the most important is this: $A\beta42$ is very sticky to itself, whereas $A\beta40$ is not. If a lot of $A\beta42$ molecules are around, they will form clumpy aggregates, almost as if they had spot-glue on their surfaces. Since this $A\beta42$ is pushed outside the cell, these clumps will form their aggregates away from the neuron.

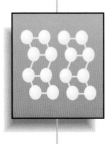

FACT #2: THE STICKINESS IS ORDERLY

$A\beta42$ molecules can stick together in a variety of ways. One way is amazingly organized, with the clumps forming orderly, compact structures. Scientists call these ordered structures *pleated sheets*, as shown on the left. They call the group of molecules in the sheet an organized fibril, rather than a disorganized clump. These fibrils are quite compact and require great amounts of $A\beta42$ to form correctly. Since the cell normally doesn't make $A\beta42$ in large quantities, these fibrils are not normally seen in the brains of healthy individuals.

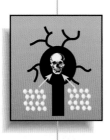

FACT #3: THE STICKINESS IS DEADLY

It is fortunate that normal cells do not make very much $A\beta42$. The reason is both interesting and frightening. It has been discovered that when $A\beta42$ forms the orderly pleated sheet discussed above, an extraordinary thing occurs: THE NEURONS SURROUNDING THE FIBRIL START DYING. The clump is actually toxic to the nerve cells! If a healthy brain started making lots of $A\beta42$, there would be a lot of cell death. Since healthy brains don't make lots of $A\beta42$, our nerve cells remain intact.

Aβ42

With these three facts in mind, we are ready to talk about Alzheimer's disease

Aβ42

When scientists first started examining the insides of plaques in Alzheimer's patients, you recall they found only the Aβ42 protein. And there were dead nerve cells surrounding the plaques. Upon close inspection, the scientists realized that many of the Aβ42-laden plaques were organized into the toxic pleated sheet forms discussed on the previous page. The following hypothesis was formulated:

Aβ42

Aβ42

People with Alzheimer's were creating much more Aβ42 than they should.

Aβ42

Remember, Aβ42 is supposed to be only a minor by-product of the cleavage of the APP protein. But the more Aβ42 made, the more likely it will form those toxic fibrils. This hypothesis has been confirmed, as shown on the graph. The data suggest that one way people can acquire Alzheimer's disease is to make more of the Aβ42 than normal.

Aβ42

Aβ42

AMOUNTS OF Aβ42 IN UNAFFECTED AND DISEASED INDIVIDUALS

Aβ42

Aβ42

The next question is: Why do Alzheimer's patients make more Aβ42 than normal? The answer appears to have been found, and it all has to do with the original APP gene. We will explain this answer more thoroughly on the next page.

Aβ42

Aβ42

Aβ42

Aβ42

Aβ42

Aβ42

PEOPLE WITH NO ALZHEIMER'S

PEOPLE WITH ALZHEIMER'S

The role of mutations

Genetic mutations are involved in the creation of the plaques found in Alzheimer's disease. Here's a review of mutations and their role in plaque formation.

On the previous page, we discovered that many Alzheimer's patients make toxic levels of the protein Aβ42. The more this protein is present, the more nerve cell damage appears to occur. On these pages, we want to ask the following question concerning these toxic levels of Aβ42:

WHY DO ALZHEIMER'S PATIENTS MAKE MORE LEVELS OF Aβ42 THAN THEY SHOULD?

To understand the answer, we will need to review some basic biology about mutations, those obnoxious mistakes in genes we discussed earlier. Then we will return to our analogy of Daddy's tailor, using him to illustrate a principle about how such mutations relate to the disease.

A As you recall, genes encode the information necessary to make proteins. Proteins are composed of tiny subunits called amino acids. There can be many thousands of amino acids in one protein.

B Like proteins, genes are also made of small subunits. These subunits are termed nucleotides, symbolized by the letters A, G, T, and C. A single gene may also have many thousands of nucleotides.

C Each group of three nucleotides codes for one particular amino acid. We call the information embedded within the gene the genetic code.

A mutation occurs if something happens to one or more of those nucleotides. A letter might be changed, for example, or one or more nucleotides may be deleted; there can even be additions. This isn't supposed to happen in a gene. When it does, the protein that is translated from the mutated gene is sometimes rendered useless. Or even worse, like a reprogrammed computer, the protein will sometimes change its function.

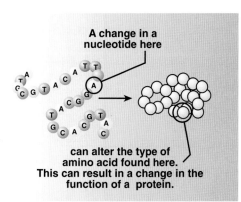

A change in a nucleotide here

can alter the type of amino acid found here. This can result in a change in the function of a protein.

MUTATIONS, AD, AND THE BUSINESS OF DADDY'S TAILOR

What do mutations have to do with Alzheimer's? As you know, Beth's father used to visit his tailor every six months to get a new suit. Just before Daddy got sick, the tailor decided to expand his shop. The tailor still made Daddy's custom suits,

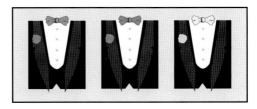

but he also began ordering mass-produced garments from a manufacturing plant. He later told Daddy that getting into mass-produced suits was the biggest mistake of his life. The reason was that many errors in manufacture were made by the plant, and he couldn't rely on the quality of the merchandise they shipped. A phone call to the plant always ended in an apology from the manager and a different excuse for the mistake, ranging from the machinery breaking down to new employees just learning the ropes. The end result was always the same, however: the suits that arrived were substandard. The tailor eventually got out of the production line of business and went back to his familiar custom work.

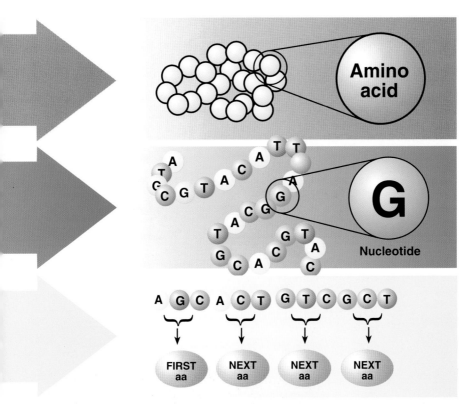

WHAT THIS HAS TO DO WITH ALZHEIMER'S

This event in the life of the tailor's business illustrates a principle needed to understand Alzheimer's disease: there can be multiple reasons for a single unsatisfactory result. With Alzheimer's, mutations or changes in function in at least four separate genes ALL appear to cause increased levels of Aβ42. Each of these genes is unique, and in a very real sense, their presence separates AD into different categories. The result is the same, however, regardless of the gene. If any of the four are mutated, the brain receives an elevated level of Aβ42. The names of these four genes, and a brief explanation of how their mutations work, are listed on the next page.

Genes associated with plaque

A number of genes are involved in the creation of the plaques found in Alzheimer's disease. Here's what we know so far.

On the last page, we mentioned that mutations in four separate genes can all lead to increased Aβ42 levels and, apparently, to disease. As shown on this page, the genes are very different from each other. The age of disease onset varies with the gene in question, for example. They all exist on separate chromosomes. Even within a single gene class, there can be many different kinds of mutations. What is so remarkable about these results is that so many different sources can all lead to the same unhappy result, an idea not unfamiliar to Daddy's tailor with his mass-produced suits. Here is a description of the four genes.

APP gene

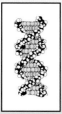

This gene should look familiar to you. It is the original APP whose protein is normally cleaved into the Aβ40 and Aβ42 fragments. For reasons not at all clear, mutations in this gene can elevate the levels of both Aβ40 and Aβ42, or just Aβ42 alone.

apoE4 gene

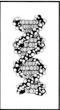

The apoE4 gene is the first gene isolated that could be used to predict if a person was going to get AD (though there is some controversy about this). The rule is this: within limits, the more copies of this gene inherited, the more likely it is that the person will get AD.* This gene is involved in an increase in the density of plaque deposits as well.

AGE OF ONSET

The kind of Alzheimer's disease a person experiences depends in part on which gene is mutated. This can be easily seen by examining the age of disease onset associated with each gene. The chart on the right illustrates in red the ages when the disease is first diagnosed and which gene is associated with which age of onset.

	0 yrs	10 yrs
APP gene		
apoE4		
Presenilin 1		
Presenilin 2		

Note: Unlike the other genes in this list, apoE4 is also associated with the sporadic form (as well as the familial form) of the disease.

CHROMOSOMAL LOCATION

Even though all four genes cause similar symptoms, they are located on very different chromosomes. As you recall from high school, human genetic information is embedded into our chromosomes (in fact, a gene is just a short segment of a chromosome). Humans have 23 pairs of chromosomes which, as shown on the right, can look like little Xs. This chart indicates which chromosome carries which AD-related gene.

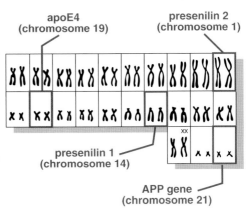

apoE4 (chromosome 19)

presenilin 2 (chromosome 1)

presenilin 1 (chromosome 14)

APP gene (chromosome 21)

Presenilin 1

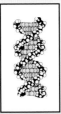

The protein encoded by this gene is embedded in the surface of the cell, looking something like a sea serpent swimming in the water. Over thirty different mutations have been described in this gene and its cousin, shown on the right. They both lead to increased levels of Aβ42.

Presenilin 2

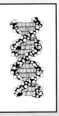

This gene is the most recently isolated sequence shown to be involved with Alzheimer's. This protein also has a serpentine look. And it tends to acquire mutations in the same place as presenilin 1, a clustering of mistakes leading to elevated Aβ42 amounts.

yrs	30 yrs	40 yrs	50 yrs	60 yrs	70 yrs

Note: Alzheimer's is often erroneously thought to be a disease of the retirement years, striking only in old age. As shown here, the disease can occur much earlier than age 65.

A problem of tangles

Amyloid plaques are not the only odd features seen in the brains of Alzheimer's patients. Structures inside the neurons, often called tangles, are also observed.

2/9/90

Bill actually asked me to dinner! That had to be some kind of first. I think he wanted me to meet Rachel, who has to be about the classiest girlfriend he's ever had. So I accepted his invitation and we had a lovely time. She really is a nurse, a bit on the heavy side, but very sweet. I can't for the life of me understand what she sees in him.

While we were chatting, I glanced at a pile of books on the living room floor, which happened to be Daddy's medical books—the stuff he has been so concerned about lately. I told Bill to bring the books to the house in a few days, and that prompted Rachel to start telling us about what's going on with Daddy's head. It was one of those lectures she promised. Rachel said what the doctors had said, that Daddy's nerve cells have gone crazy, spitting out weird molecule-things which act like glue, gumming up Daddy's ability to think. She also said that the insides of his nerves have really strange things happening inside them too—with the same effect as the stuff on the outside. I didn't understand much after that, so I'm thinking of asking her out for coffee. I wonder if she'd be willing to continue her chat.

In her discussion of what Beth termed in her journal "molecule-things which act like glue," Rachel was describing the presence of the amyloid plaques, and we have been talking about the genes responsible for their creation. As we've seen, however, the plaques first noticed by Dr. Alzheimer were not the only odd structures in the brains of Alzheimer's patients. He also observed structures he called "tangles." To get a fuller picture of the molecules behind AD, we will spend the next few pages talking about these tangles. The internal tangles were noted in Rachel's description to Beth and Bill—and are described more fully below.

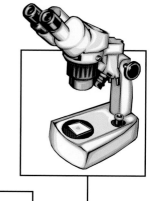

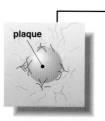

plaque

Dr. Alzheimer's observations included looking at structures on both the outside and inside of nerve cells. He found that the amyloid plaques were invariably located outside nerve cells. But he consistently noticed another odd structure that lay on the inside of nerve cells. These structures consisted of highly ordered parallel lines, looking like bundles of sticks. He also noticed that they appeared to outlast the nerve cells that carried them. Even when the rest of the cell disappeared, the parallel bundles still remained. These bundles are now called neurofibrillary tangles.

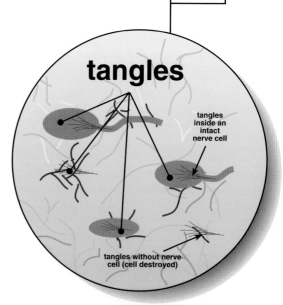

tangles

tangles inside an intact nerve cell

tangles without nerve cell (cell destroyed)

A SKELETON FOR NERVE CELLS

To understand what neurofibrillary tangles have to do with AD, we need to discuss some of the internal anatomy of a nerve cell. We'll begin with a few comments on overall structure. It might surprise you to learn that the cells in your body possess a tiny skeleton, just as the rest of your body possesses a large skeleton. As shown in the picture below, this extraordinary feature of our cells is called a *cytoskeleton*, and it is a very complex structure.

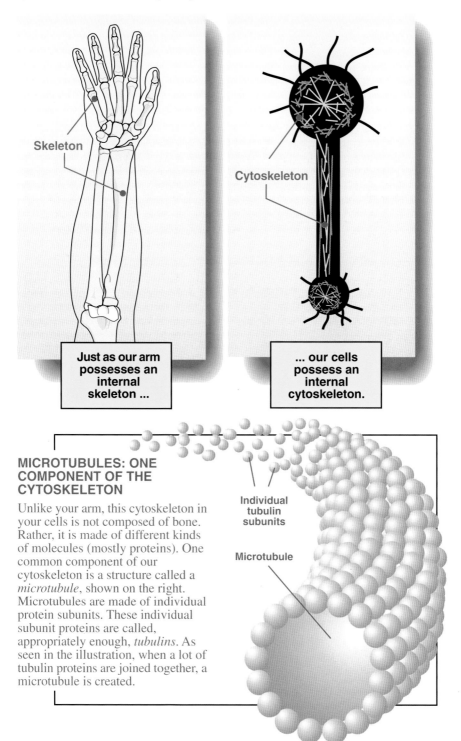

Skeleton

Cytoskeleton

Just as our arm possesses an internal skeleton ...

... our cells possess an internal cytoskeleton.

MICROTUBULES: ONE COMPONENT OF THE CYTOSKELETON

Unlike your arm, this cytoskeleton in your cells is not composed of bone. Rather, it is made of different kinds of molecules (mostly proteins). One common component of our cytoskeleton is a structure called a *microtubule*, shown on the right. Microtubules are made of individual protein subunits. These individual subunit proteins are called, appropriately enough, *tubulins*. As seen in the illustration, when a lot of tubulin proteins are joined together, a microtubule is created.

Individual tubulin subunits

Microtubule

The tau of AD

Tangles are made from specific molecules.
One protein found in tangles is called tau.

As you know, the goal of this book is to explain what happens to the brain affeted by Alzheimer's disease. Because it is a biological disorder, we needed to review some basic science to understand just how it all works. Perhaps, like Beth wrote in her journal, you have not been used to reading a lot of complex science. Rest assured, we are nearing the end of our discussion of the "whys" of AD, and must tackle only one more subject. To realize how tangles are involved in AD, we will talk about some of the roles microtubules play in the functioning of a normal nerve cell, as well as in Alzheimer's disease.

2/13/90

Bill's girlfriend actually took me up on my offer to chat—will miracles never cease?—and today we went out for coffee. I thought Rachel was going to ask me about my brother, and was I ready to give her an earful! But that's not what we talked about at all. Instead, we talked almost the whole time about Daddy. She seemed very concerned about me burning out, and showed much more interest in what was going on with Daddy than Bill ever did. Rachel even had Daddy's books with her, which she returned sheepishly. But she had marked some areas that she thought I might have been interested in, especially concerning our conversation of a couple of days ago. It was all about what was going on with the cells in Daddy's head. I promised I would read them, though to be perfectly honest, that was a lie. I never could understand anything in Daddy's books.

MORE ON MICROTUBULES

Microtubules are really extraordinary structures. They are not rigid and stiff like a bone. Rather, microtubules are fluid, constantly forming at one end and disassembling at the other. This provides a tremendous amount of flexibility that allows them to supervise some of the cell's most important functions. Three of these functions are listed below.

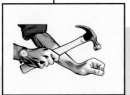

STRUCTURE. Microtubules form a network with other molecules to provide shape and form to a cell. Even though they are flexible by nature, microtubules work like a pliable scaffolding. As such, they are something like our skeletons. Without microtubules, the cell would lose its characteristic structure, a disaster for cells like neurons.

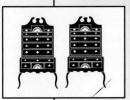

COMPARTMENTALIZATION. A normal cell needs to demarcate certain internal areas to perform specific functions. We call these areas microcompartments, and their existence is critical to the life of a cell. Microtubules are used to divide the cell's interior into specific sections, something like wood is used to create drawers in a dresser.

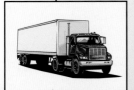

TRANSPORT. Microtubules also provide internal transport for certain important molecules. Different regions within the interior require specific molecules in order to function. Microtubules work something like trucks driving across town with full loads. The fact that microtubules are dynamic, assembling and disassembling, allows this transport to occur.

DON'T THEY NEED HELP?

Microtubules have a lot of work to do in a typical nerve cell, many more functions than just the three listed on the previous page. With all that work to do, you might expect that microtubules could use some assistance. And the cell provides such help. There are many accessory proteins that work with microtubules, collectively called MAPs (short for *microtubule-associated proteins*) to assist them in their various chores.

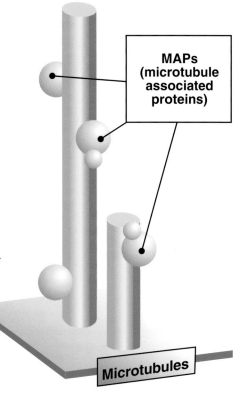

One important MAP—especially as it relates to AD—is a protein that goes by the odd name of *tau*. Tau works with microtubules in nerve cells three ways: first, it helps to stabilize their structure, thus aiding in shape; secondly, it assists microtubules in the establishment of various microcompartments; thirdly, tau helps facilitate the transport of various molecules from one part of the nerve cell to the next. As you can imagine, tau is very important in the overall functioning of a nerve cell. Without tau, the microtubules would fall apart and the cell would die. A graphical representation of MAPs such as tau is shown in the drawing on the right.

WHAT ABOUT THE TANGLES?

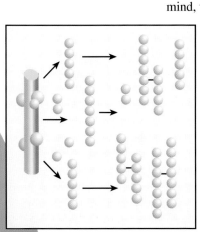

With some of the organization of microtubules in mind, we are ready to return to Alzheimer's disease and the tangles seen in nerve cells. As you recall, these tangles are actually linear filaments, looking something like sticks that have been bound together. One of the first questions scientists asked, naturally, was "What are tangles made of?" The answer they received was astonishing. *The tangles contained the tau protein.* The very same protein sprinkled along the microtubules in nerve cells! But the tau proteins weren't randomly sprinkled across microtubules any more. Rather, the tau proteins were adhering to each other, forming stick-like structures, and then the sticks started binding together to form the tangles. The questions, of course, were manifold, such as: Why did the tau abandon their normal job? What made them form into the sticklike filaments? And *then,* what made the filaments bind together to form the characteristic tangles?

A change in tau's function

Understanding tangle formation involves explaining why tau changes its function inside nerve cells. Here's a review of what we know so far.

As we discovered on the last page, the tangles found in Alzheimer's nerve cells are made of the protein tau. This important molecule normally interacts with microtubules, providing assistance in cell shape and internal transport. These functions are so important that if tau is ever destroyed, or even disrupted, the nerve cell will die. When enough nerve cells die in the brain, the organ can no longer function correctly. Memory loss is observed, as is the odd behavior. The more tangles, the more severe the symptoms of Alzheimer's become. As you might expect, finding out why tau changes its job description and starts forming tangles inside nerves is a very important question in Alzheimer's research.

Perhaps incredibly, the questions posed both here and on the previous page are beginning to be answered. The insight appears to come from a biological process we have not yet covered in detail. To understand how the protein tau changes its function, and what that has to do with AD, we will need to review briefly a process that occurs some time after the tau protein is made. And to do that, we shall return one last time to the metaphor of the tailor from whom Daddy bought his new suits. This involves some of his custom work.

A LAST VISIT TO THE TAILOR

Daddy's tailor knew that the good doctor was a fussy, no-nonsense customer. Daddy was also quite detail-oriented, and insisted on seeing the stitching and cuffs, even the color of buttons, that were going onto the suit he ordered. He was especially fond of vests, the kind that was belted in the back. Being a good-natured tailor, he allowed Daddy the freedom to design. After the fabric was cut, both men would decide what kinds of buttons and buckles, even zippers, to place on the suit. And then the tailor would finish the job.

What does the placement of accessories have to do with human molecules, specifically tau proteins? There are mechanisms deep within our cells that work a lot like Daddy's tailor. After the protein is made and cut, the cell often puts "accessories" on the newly formed molecule—just like the tailor might put buttons on a vest. But the accessories that are placed on these proteins are not plastic; they are instead tiny little molecules. You may even be familiar with some of them. One molecule that is frequently placed on proteins is called a phosphate group, the same kind of phosphate often found in laundry detergent. Another molecule that is often placed on newly formed proteins is a type of sugar.

Just as buttons are placed on the finished jacket,	so can small molecules be placed on a new protein.

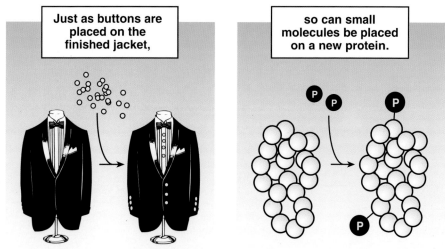

WHAT HAPPENS WHEN A SMALL MOLECULE IS ADDED?

The cell has to be very careful about how and where it places its small accessory molecules. The reason is simple: the addition often changes the function of the protein that gets it. If many phosphates are placed onto a protein when it only should get a few, for example, the protein may start behaving very differently. The same thing is true with sugars. As we shall see, the addition of such accessories plays a great role in changing the function of tau.

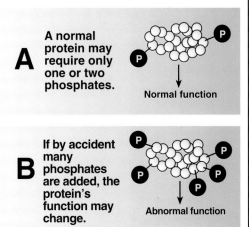

A A normal protein may require only one or two phosphates.

Normal function

B If by accident many phosphates are added, the protein's function may change.

Abnormal function

WHAT DOES THIS HAVE TO DO WITH TANGLES?

As you know, we are trying to answer questions like: what causes tau proteins to change their function, to start adhering to each other, forming stick-like structures? And then, what causes those sticks to form the bundles we know as tangles? The answer has to do with the accessories the tau protein acquires.

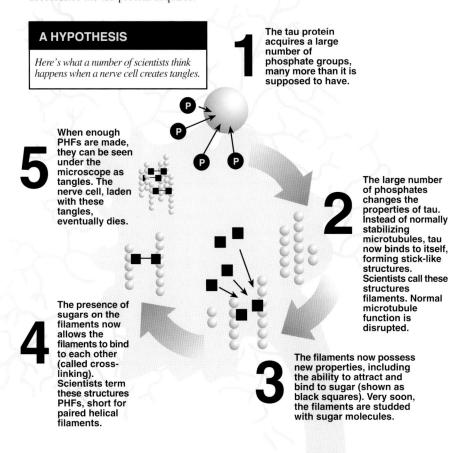

A HYPOTHESIS

Here's what a number of scientists think happens when a nerve cell creates tangles.

1 The tau protein acquires a large number of phosphate groups, many more than it is supposed to have.

2 The large number of phosphates changes the properties of tau. Instead of normally stabilizing microtubules, tau now binds to itself, forming stick-like structures. Scientists call these structures filaments. Normal microtubule function is disrupted.

3 The filaments now possess new properties, including the ability to attract and bind to sugar (shown as black squares). Very soon, the filaments are studded with sugar molecules.

4 The presence of sugars on the filaments now allows the filaments to bind to each other (called cross-linking). Scientists term these structures PHFs, short for paired helical filaments.

5 When enough PHFs are made, they can be seen under the microscope as tangles. The nerve cell, laden with these tangles, eventually dies.

As you can see, the addition of both phosphates and sugars changes tau enough that the protein turns toxic. There is a great deal of work attempting to discover why tau gets too many phosphates and sugars. In many ways, these questions represent the cutting edge of Alzheimer's research today.

A review of the chapter

From plaques to tangles, we have gone over a large amount of biology in this chapter. Here is a quick review of some of the topics we discussed.

We have attempted here to answer the "why" questions of Alzheimer's disease. As we have seen, this is not easy to do. It turns out that there are many Alzheimer's diseases, with very different origins. Even with these advances, we have mostly explored the familial type, representing about 5% of all the cases reported in this country. It is hoped that the clues discovered with the familial type will someday shed light on the other 95%. Shown below are some of the topics we covered in our attempt to better understand the effects of this disease on human brains.

ABOUT PLAQUES

Basic Biology

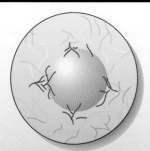

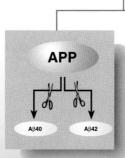

PLAQUES
Plaques are spherelike structures existing just outside nerve cells. Called senile plaques by Dr. Alzheimer, they are surrounded by degenerating axon terminals and dendrite branches.

APP GENE
Short for amyloid precursor protein, this molecule can be cleaved into two smaller proteins. One such product, called Aβ42, was found to be a major component of senile plaques.

MUTATIONS
To understand plaque formation, we needed to explore the concept of genetic mutation. Mutations are mistakes in the genetic code, errors that can be passed on to their proteins.

ABOUT TANGLES

Basic Biology

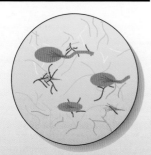

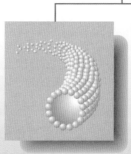

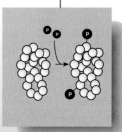

TANGLES
Tangles are abnormal structures found inside the nerve cells of Alzheimer's patients. They are highly ordered bundles of molecules that can kill the nerve cells in which they reside.

CYTOSKELETON
To understand tangles and AD, it was important to know about the cytoskeleton found in nerve cells. This complex collection of molecules works like the large skeleton in the human body.

SMALL MOLECULES
We also needed to know that cellular proteins can be modified by the addition of small molecules. Two common molecules that can be added are phosphate groups and sugars.

IS IT AS SIMPLE AS PLAQUES AND TANGLES?

The answer, of course, is no. The mechanisms reviewed below, while fairly well-understood, do not address all the issues surrounding the origins of this disease. Nor do they explain all the data regarding the presence or absence of symptoms already well-established. As we have mentioned, nerve-destroying plaques have been found in people who showed no outward signs of disease (the tangles seem to be a better sign as to the intensity of the disease—the more there are, the more severe the symptoms). There are other data regarding origins of AD which have to do with mechanisms like strokes, aluminum and something called oxidative stress. Some of these are described in the appendix in the back of this book. But all of them will have to be integrated into the data presented in this chapter to get a complete picture of this debilitating disease.

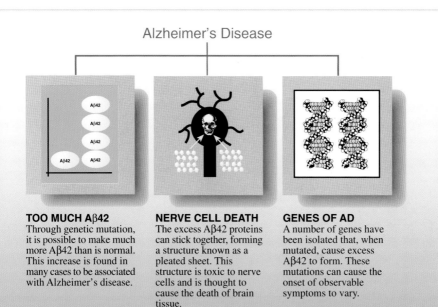

TOO MUCH Aβ42
Through genetic mutation, it is possible to make much more Aβ42 than is normal. This increase is found in many cases to be associated with Alzheimer's disease.

NERVE CELL DEATH
The excess Aβ42 proteins can stick together, forming a structure known as a pleated sheet. This structure is toxic to nerve cells and is thought to cause the death of brain tissue.

GENES OF AD
A number of genes have been isolated that, when mutated, cause excess Aβ42 to form. These mutations can cause the onset of observable symptoms to vary.

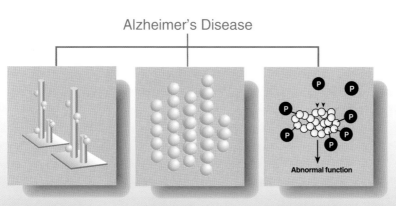

TAU PROTEINS
To know the relevance of these small additions to proteins, we needed to describe microtubules. These cylindrical structures have molecules associated with them. One such protein is called tau.

FILAMENTS
Under certain conditions, tau proteins will form stick-like structures. Called filaments, these aggregated tau proteins can form into tangles; neurons containing them eventually die.

MODIFICATION
The reason tau proteins change their normal function involves modification by small molecules. Both phosphates and sugars are thought to be involved.

how

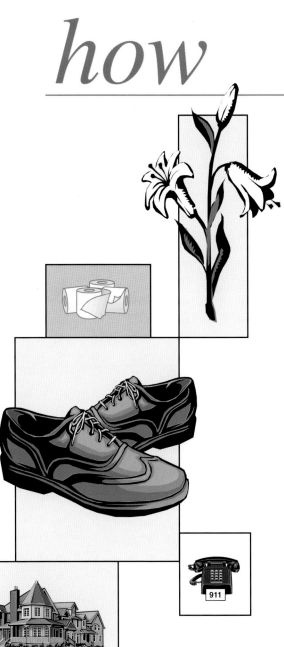

caring for the Alzheimer's patient: practical suggestions

- *General principles in caring for persons with Alzheimer's disease*

- *How to deal with difficult behavior*

- *Coping with specific kinds of memory loss*

- *Securing the living quarters*

- *Dealing with meals and mealtime*

- *Personal hygiene*

- *Dealing with urinary and fecal incontinence*

- *Exercise and recreation*

- *Planning for the end*

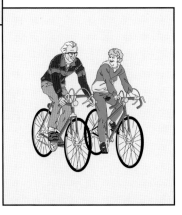

Dealing with the everyday issues

In this last part of the book, we discuss how to care for a person with AD.

This section is dedicated to the "hows" of caring for an Alzheimer's patient. In the first section we discussed the "whats" of AD, looking at common behaviors experienced by people with the disorder. The next section was devoted to the "whys" of Alzheimer's, seeking to understand both the biology of the brain and the kinds of molecules that create the disease. In this last part, we will use the knowledge gathered from the previous two sections to address the very human issues of caring for someone who is progressively losing the use of many brain functions.

Implicit in this discussion is the idea that the mind of an adult is lost only in pieces. It must be remembered that people with AD remain very human adults, complete with an ability to become bewildered, humiliated, loved and appreciated, even though they are suffering progressive brain damage. Moreover, AD sometimes allows its patients to appear to "flicker" back to normal, more familiar behavior. This imparts a cruel reminder of just how human a person is, even when burdened with plaques and tangles.

Consider one of Beth's entries in her diary, a paragraph written three years after Daddy was diagnosed.

1/24/90

It's like a scab that gets picked off every two weeks. Daddy soiled his pants last night just before the ten o'clock news. But an hour later, I caught him downstairs, furiously pounding on his old electric typewriter. When I asked him what he was doing, he looked at me like I haven't seen him in almost 3 years—calm, collected, even matter-of-fact. And then something incredible happened. He actually called my name! He said "Hello, Beth." This morning, Daddy was back in Alzheimer's land again, shouting for the umpteenth time for my long-deceased mother. When I went down to see what he had typed the night before, I couldn't understand it. Not because it was gibberish. It was some kind of new idea for a surgical technique he apparently had been thinking about. I couldn't believe the man that was shouting in my house this morning was the same one who was working so hard last night!

This entry in Beth's journal is just another way of saying that a person with Alzheimer's is still a human being— and an adult human being at that. It also underscores the fact that AD isn't a fault, nor a form of stubbornness, nor a plunge into immaturity. AD is a disease as surely as diabetes is a disease; that it afflicts the organ that governs our behavior does not make it any less physical.

Such a point of view provides clues as to how caregivers should react to a given patient at various stages of disease. In this chapter we are going to explore some of those clues, describing a few general principles about caregiving for a person with Alzheimer's. In the next chapter, we will relate these general principles to specific issues of living daily with AD, such as coping with memory loss or supervising a loved one's personal hygiene.

We begin our journey of integrating caregiving and biology by reexamining the brain of an Alzheimer's patient. Attempts have been made to link the behavioral progression of the disease with the timing of brain damage. Shown below is a model published in the *British Journal of Nursing*, associating what is seen by the caregiver with what occurs within the patient's brain.

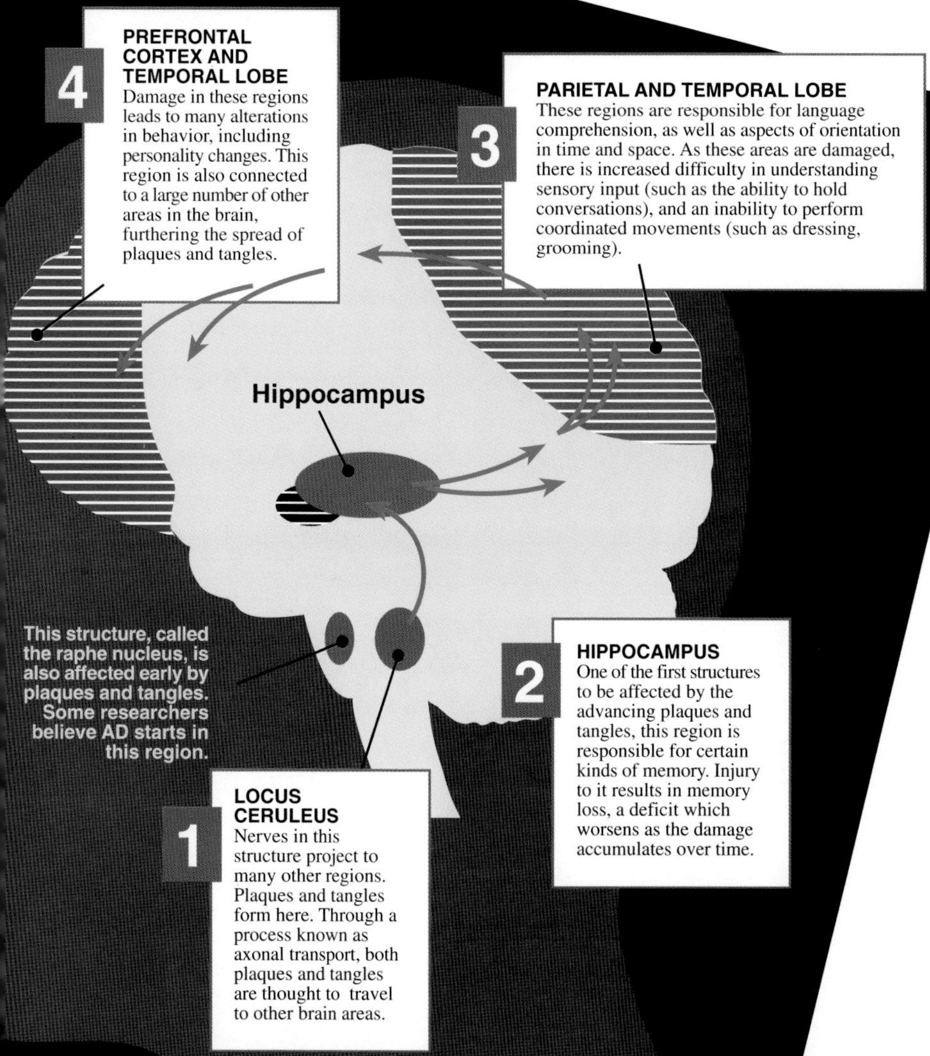

4

PREFRONTAL CORTEX AND TEMPORAL LOBE
Damage in these regions leads to many alterations in behavior, including personality changes. This region is also connected to a large number of other areas in the brain, furthering the spread of plaques and tangles.

3

PARIETAL AND TEMPORAL LOBE
These regions are responsible for language comprehension, as well as aspects of orientation in time and space. As these areas are damaged, there is increased difficulty in understanding sensory input (such as the ability to hold conversations), and an inability to perform coordinated movements (such as dressing, grooming).

Hippocampus

This structure, called the raphe nucleus, is also affected early by plaques and tangles. Some researchers believe AD starts in this region.

2

HIPPOCAMPUS
One of the first structures to be affected by the advancing plaques and tangles, this region is responsible for certain kinds of memory. Injury to it results in memory loss, a deficit which worsens as the damage accumulates over time.

1

LOCUS CERULEUS
Nerves in this structure project to many other regions. Plaques and tangles form here. Through a process as known as axonal transport, both plaques and tangles are thought to travel to other brain areas.

OTHER PATHS

Many aspects of the pattern drawn above need further experimental verification to be considered fact. One neural pathway researchers *have* shown to be deeply involved in AD is called the cholinergic pathway. This pathway is a set of associated neurons that use acetylcholine as their neurotransmitter, and are projected throughout the brain. Certain researchers believe that parts of this pathway are devastated early in the progress of the disease.

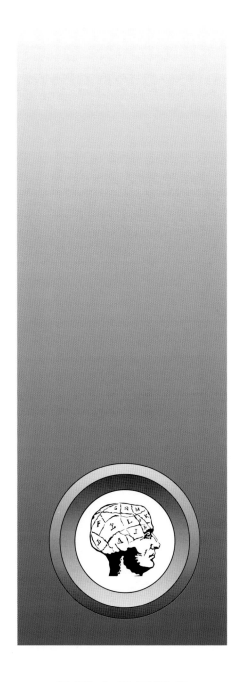

CHAPTER
SIX

*Caring for the
Alzheimer's patient*

Principles of caring for people with Alzheimer's disease

Understanding the biology of Alzheimer's disease allows us to create a framework for the care and managment of people who have it. Here are a few key principles.

Attempting to provide meaningful suggestions to the caregiver of someone progressing through AD is understandably difficult. While science has revealed to us the biological nature of the disease, no two people experience AD the same way. Thus, it may be most helpful to relate general principles about caring based on common experience. These pages attempt to do just that, beginning with some observations about human behavior, then speculating as to how a person with AD may view the world and the caregiver's efforts to help.

two principles and a matter of timing

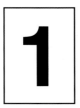

THE POWER OF CONTEXT

Behavior never occurs in a vacuum, whether someone has AD or not. For better or worse, people usually do what makes sense to them. Thus behaviors must always be understood in context, which leads to the hope that they have meaning and may be understood. This includes behaviors related to AD. In attempting to modify the negative behaviors of their patients, caregivers can learn which approaches are successful and which are not.

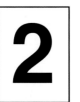

THE LOSS OF CONTROL

Some negative behaviors of people with AD will occur despite a caregiver's best attempts to minimize environmental triggers. A patient's actions may make no obvious sense to anyone, perhaps not even to the afflicted person. Even this has a context, however puzzling it may be. The most complex organ in the world is undergoing a selective deterioration whose damage cannot be predicted with current technology. There will thus be times when the only understanding of an AD person's behavior is that it will not be understandable.

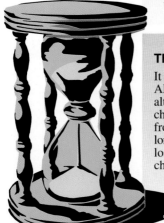

THE IMPORTANCE OF TIMING

It is important to remember that many behaviors of AD patients will change over time. Two kinds of alterations are observed. There are short-term changes,where a person varies specific behaviors from day to day, even hour to hour. There are also long-term changes, where an alteration or a particular loss of function becomes permanent. The kinds of changes observed depend upon the person, and no one can precisely predict which changes will occur or when they will be observed.

SOMEONE ELSE'S SHOES

One of the most important keys to knowing how to care for a person with AD comes directly from the patient. A specific behavior, while potentially difficult to interpret, may carry with it an understandable message if the caregiver can decipher what is being communicated. How can such decoding take place? The old adage that says that you cannot understand a person unless you have walked a mile in his shoes may have some relevance here. Written below are descriptions of feelings many Alzheimer's patients have as they experience the disease. Understanding the world through their perspective can yield vital clues to the appropriate reaction for the caregiver.

FRUSTRATIONS

As their brains deteriorate, the world of the person with Alzheimer's disease begins to turn upside down. Understandably, they may react to such changes the way you might, with fear, frustration, even anger. As further damage occurs, an AD patient may become overwhelmed with stimulation, or recoil at their world when suddenly nothing looks familiar. They may issue complex, repetitive demands in an attempt to "regroup" or "reorganize."

FOR EXAMPLE

Mrs. Loren, a widow living with her adult son, woke up from a nap quite suddenly. She ran into the den and shouted to her son, "I want my husband. I want him right now! Get him for me!" For what seemed to be the millionth time, her son tried to explain that her husband was dead. Ten minutes later, Mrs. Loren again walked into the den and demanded to know where her husband was.

SENSITIVITIES

People with AD often become hypersensitive to nonverbal communcation. If the caregiver is agitated, frustrated or harsh, the caregiver may attempt to cover with soothing words. This can backfire. The person with AD will often respond not to what is being said, but to the body language and the tone being perceived. Additionally, they are very sensitive to their environment and to demands made of them. They are much less likely to exhibit negative, destructive behavior if they are in relaxing, familiar settings with predictable routines and requests contoured to their remaining capacities.

FOR EXAMPLE

John almost exploded when his regular caregiver called in sick and a substitute was sent. She wasn't very experienced, and even though her voice seemed reassuring, John could tell she was nervous. When his meal was late, John began yelling at her, demanding that his normal cargiver return.

FEARS AND FAILURES

Alzheimer's patients, like anyone, fear failure and embarrassment. As their world continues to spin out of control, they may begin to resist activities they sense are too difficult. It must also be remembered that people with AD are still adults, even if their behavior sometimes speaks otherwise. They are thus very sensitive to a patronizing reaction, to a demeaning tone of voice, to baby talk, or being ignored and discussed as if they aren't there. They may additionally resist tasks they consider degrading.

FOR EXAMPLE

Eighty-year-old Eloise started receiving in-home nursing assistance. One day, an aide named Cameron commented at how "cute" Eloise looked in her "fuzzy little slippers." Eloise became suddenly tearful, and started backing away from Cameron, eventually retreating to the bathroom. It took him all afternoon to persuade Eloise to come out.

EFFORTS AND ATTITUDES

Most AD patients, especially in the initial stages, know something is terribly wrong. They try as hard as they can to correct what is amiss, an attitude that may not change until the very late stages of the disease. Trying to reason with them as their brains deteriorate, or arguing, pleading, even punishing them for their behavior, will not make them get well. It may only make them become more frustrated with something over which they have no control, and would themselves get rid of if they could.

FOR EXAMPLE

Try as he might, Ted had an extremely difficult time understanding his ailing dad's reactions. Sometimes his father would just cry and cry in his rocking chair. Ted would catch him trying to read an old letter, get angry and throw the letter down. "I can't, I can't, I can't," was all his dad would say. Ted lost patience with this one day, practically yelling for his father to tell him what "I can't" meant. He would only grow silent.

How to deal with difficult behavior: Part I

The hardest part about caregiving can be learning the correct responses to difficult, even bizarre behavior. Listed below are a few principles that may help.

In the last page, we suggested that the unfamiliar conduct of AD patients may have reasons and contexts, and that this perspective gives hints to help caregivers in their hardest task: responding to difficult behaviors. These hints have been organized into a number of general principles useful for caregivers and outlined in the next four pages. As always, it is important to remember that not everyone will experience Alzheimer's in exactly the same way; patients are quite likely to show different patterns of behavior as the disease progresses. These principles are thus meant to serve as flexible suggestions, applicable to a variety of difficult behaviors caregivers are likely to encounter.

REASSURE

Security issues can play a major role in the emotional turmoil many Alzheimer's patients exhibit. One powerful tool for addressing such behaviors is reassurance, addressed to an AD patient whose world increasingly slips from her grasp. A caregiver can remind the patient that she is not isolated and forgotten, but rather valued and loved. Such reassurance can be used to reinstill a sense of security that the patient will be protected from harm and even from embarrassment. Hugs or just staying around her general vicinity may be useful in communicating such security.

REDIRECT

It is possible to alter difficult behavior by redirecting it into a different, perhaps more positive, activity. Someone who constantly rummages through drawers in a dresser may be given a specific organizing task, such as sorting out buttons in a sewing drawer, or wrapping loose coins in a coin jacket. A restless, distraught person may be directed to rake old leaves or sweep out the garage. Distracting the person may be useful as well. Going for a ride, putting on a favorite video, introducing snacks or other treats and otherwise redirecting a patient's focus may be helpful.

RESTRUCTURE

As the AD patient's world careens out of control, it may be important to restructure daily rituals to accommodate the patient's best time of day—and then keep to the schedule. Creating predictable routines is a great way to foster temporal security. In many cases, the key ingredient for creating reassurance is repetition. Determining a pleasant activity and then repeating it often may involve rearranging the day, but it may also provide a more secure framework. Pleasant activities may include reading favorite stories, hearing or singing favorite songs, looking over old photographs, etc.

RETHINK

Part of learning to respond to difficult behavior means adjusting the attitudes of the caregiver. The stark reality of Alzheimer's is that unusual behavior often occurs for no discernible reason; sometimes no amount of reassuring, redirecting, or restructuring will help. Instead, a caregiver may ask himself questions such as "Can I increase my tolerance for the bizarre behaviors?" Another question the caregiver must ask is "Can I modify my expectations?" Such changes in attitudes are sometimes the only response a caregiver can give as the patient continues to deteriorate. At these times, it is often wise for caregivers to seek emotional support and counseling from outside sources.

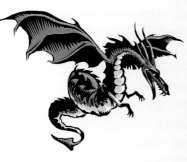

AVOIDING A CATASTROPHIC REACTION

An Alzheimer's patient may some times appear to "blow up." She may suddenly erupt emotionally and start screaming, throwing things or acting in an otherwise severely disruptive manner. Just as suddenly, the reaction may subside, the patient resuming her daily routine as if nothing had happened. Mental health professionals call this behavior a *catastrophic reaction*. It may come about for a variety of reasons, many of which are mentioned in this chapter. The suggestions for managing behavior are in part an attempt to avoid repeated rounds of catastrophic reactions.

4/19/90

Daddy's afternoon four o'clock wanderings and cries for Mom are driving me crazy. I called Amy and just dumped on her, bless her heart, because after all these years I still miss Mom, too. I'm glad we had the talk. In the middle of the conversation, Amy came up with a great idea about Daddy. She suggested that the next time he got goofy, especially when he mentioned Mom, that I take Daddy down to the basement. He naturally loves organization, and since he and Mom have a whole bunch of junk down there that's just lying around, Amy suggested that I give Daddy a project. Maybe he could put their things into boxes and start labeling them. I wasn't sure if that was such a good idea, thinking that digging up old memories might make him distraught. Or that even the fact it was a mess down there might cause him to freak out. But Amy pointed out that Daddy was already upset in the afternoon, and that if he got antsy, we could always stop what was going on. She has a good point there. I'm thinking maybe I will try it tomorrow.

4/20/90

I called Amy tonight and told her that she is some kind of genius. I didn't even wait for Daddy to start moaning about Mom. As soon as it was four in the afternoon, I just took him downstairs, started the cleanup and asked him to join in. He went after the cleaning project with a vengeance! Daddy was surprisingly careful—opening up old cardboard boxes, sorting through things, placing items into plastic tubs, others into the garbage. He got agitated a few times, but I found his old phonograph and some record albums that must have been released around the time Daddy and Mom were dating. I started playing them, wondering if the music would be soothing. I was anxious at first, the power of old memories and all, but I didn't need to worry. Daddy became quite calm, even smiled a time or two, and continued making great progress putting things away, which surprised me no end. I'm thinking that this would be a great activity to do in the late afternoon, when he's most likely to be goofy.

How to deal with difficult behavior: Part II

Emphasizing solutions by taking the sufferer's point of view will not always work, despite the caregiver's best intentions. Under a physician's care, it may be possible to treat certain disruptive behaviors with medications (antidepressants are sometimes given to people with AD, for example, as are medications like buspirone and valproate). How or when a person should start or stop taking medications are issues to be solved in consultation with the family doctor or other supervising medical professional (for example, a geriatric psychiatrist).

Sometimes situations require caregivers to be proactive in the way they treat their patients. Listed below are steps a caregiver can take in responding to troublesome situations, regardless of the presence or absence of medicines.

STOP THE STRESS

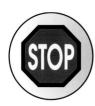

Reducing environmental stress can be a key component in responding to difficult behaviors. A person with AD can become easily agitated if his environment overstimulates him. It may be important to avoid noisy public places, for example, or to stop rushing from one place to the next when running errands. Creating environments that simplify the complex strains of life, or avoiding hyperstimulation altogether, may soothe an easily agitated person with AD, making him less prone to difficult behavior.

SUBSTITUTE

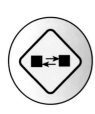

Compensating for someone's loss of function can be an important part of dealing with troublesome situations. It can be quite comforting, for example, to do specific tasks for an Alzheimer's patient that he can no longer do for himself. A caregiver may order a meal if making such a decision begins to create distress and agitation for their patient. A caregiver may discreetly carry a card in a public place that says "My companion has a memory disorder. Please direct your questions to me." Additionally, a caregiver can redirect a person with AD to a less conspicuous place if he begins to exhibit socially awkward behavior such as disrobing or masturbating in public.

SIMPLIFY

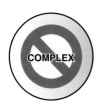

Along with making a person's environment less overwhelming, a caregiver's personal interactions with the patient may require simplification. Difficult situations can sometimes be diffused by breaking tasks into single-step, easily executed instructions. Using concrete, readily understood terms can be enormously helpful in clarifying situations and calming an agitated person (it must be kept in mind however, that while a tendency to "talk down" to a person while simplifying one's vocabulary can be great, it is important never to patronize a person with AD). Part of simplificaiton may also include taking repeated and predictable breaks from a specific task.

SOOTHE

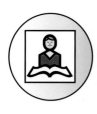

Another technique involves using specific tasks to soothe and calm. It is possible to create pleasant moments and reminisce about cherished events with a person with AD. Even if soon forgotten, the exercises can deeply affect mood and behavior. Sensory exercises can involve music, art, even physical activity. So can activities such as reviewing old pictures in a photo album, repeating favorite prayers, hymns, poems, brushing the person's hair, giving massages, and so on. Even the presentation and interaction with familiar objects, such as a favorite blanket, article of clothing, a childhood trinket, can act as a source of security for an agitated person with AD.

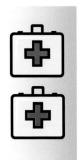

PUTTING SAFETY FIRST

One of the most difficult situations a caregiver must address comes when the patient engages in a dangerous activity. As we have previously discussed, people with AD can have the disturbing ability to wander off or lay hold of items that could potentially hurt them. It is very important to lock up guns, secure storage areas that hold toxic household chemicals (such as cleaning material) and otherwise eliminate situations of potential harm. It may even be useful to disguise exits. Additionally a person with AD can be registered in a program administered through the Alzheimer's Association called SAFE RETURN, in case the patient wanders off and gets lost (see Appendix F for addresses and phone numbers).

FOR EXAMPLE

The Nolan family used to be able to have a radio blaring in one room and a TV on in another, even when Uncle Gregory came to live with them. One day, when the rock music was particularly loud, the 15-year-old daughter found her uncle banging his head against the wall. When he saw her, he yelled something unintelligible and then began to cry. The frightened daughter reported this to her mother. From that time until the day Uncle Gregory was admitted to a nursing home, the daughter had to use headphones when she wanted to listen to the radio.

FOR EXAMPLE

Evelyn's older sister, Mary, was still able to use her knife and fork for many years after she was found to have Alzheimer's disease. One day, however, when Mary was seated at dinner, she simply stared at her pork chop. Mary ate the beans and the potatoes, but would not eat anything else. The next morning a similar thing occurred with her breakfast sausage. Evelyn eventually figured out that Mary had lost the ability to cut her own food, even though she could still hold a knife and use her spoon and fork. At dinner time, Evelyn began to serve her sister bite-sized portions of meat or, when the occasion called for it, would cut Mary's portions for her.

FOR EXAMPLE

Brian's father, who was diagnosed with Alzheimer's years ago, had a terrible time getting himself dressed. It was a fairly vigorous frustration, and Brian decided he would try to help his dad. His efforts just seemed to make matters worse, unfortunately. Brian would bark out instructions like "Put on your shirt" or "Make sure your socks match," and his dad would fumble and then start yelling. Brian eventually learned from his home care nurse to take things much more slowly. Now Brian says things like "Put your left arm through the sleeve. Now your right arm. Okay, now use the buttons ..." Dressing became much easier as a result.

FOR EXAMPLE

Diane didn't know what she was going to do about her mother's sullen behavior. She had been taking antidepressant medication for a while now, but for some reason, she had begun retreating to her room. Coming across some old pictures of her parents, Diane realized that her mom and dad had done a fair amount of ballroom dancing in their younger years. She went to a store and bought a CD of big-band standards, and then played them on the living room stereo. The first time she heard the music, her mother came walking down the hall. Diane asked her if she could "have this dance." Her mother refused shyly but, to Diane's surprise, spent the entire evening with her in the living room.

One strategy for addressing difficult behaviors

Though every caregiver encounters different and changing needs in their patients, it is possible to create a system for solving the most difficult problems.

The last few pages have been devoted to explaining principles of responding to difficult behavior. These principles can be used to create an overall strategy for solving the day-to-day challenges that come with caring for an Alzheimer's patient. This strategy is outlined as a flow chart on these pages. It assumes a specific difficult problem has arisen with a patient under the supervision of a caregiver. The first question the caregiver asks, after identifying the behavior, has to do with the potential for harm. This assessment might concern the patient or the people surrounding the patient (including the caregiver).

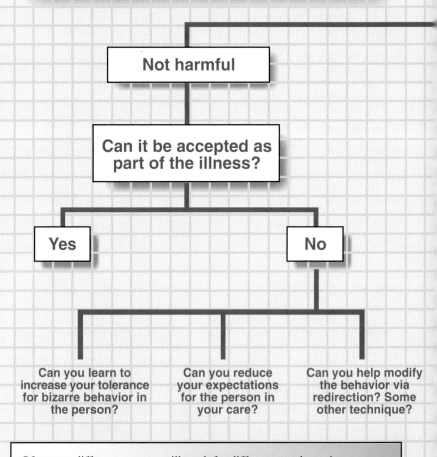

Not harmful

Can it be accepted as part of the illness?

Yes **No**

Can you learn to increase your tolerance for bizarre behavior in the person?

Can you reduce your expectations for the person in your care?

Can you help modify the behavior via redirection? Some other technique?

Of course, different systems will work for different people, and may vary for the same person at different stages in the disease. This strategy, as well as the principles outlined in this chapter, are meant only as suggestions to assist caregivers as they seek to form a routine for their patients. In addition to these ideas, there are a number of considerations that can help address specific problems of daily living and care for a person with AD. Some of these more practical suggestions are described in the next chapter.

What is the problem?

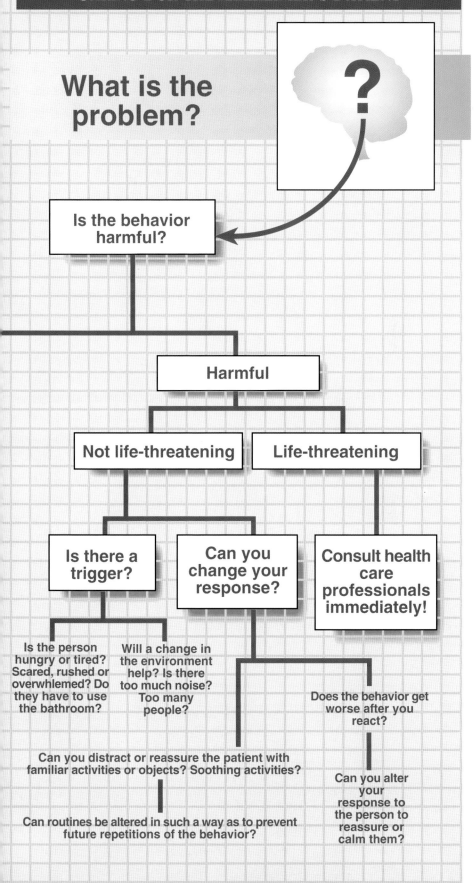

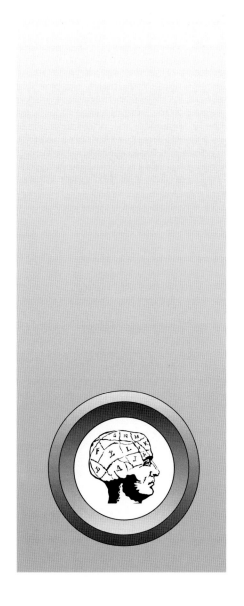

CHAPTER
SEVEN

*Living with Alzheimer's:
practical suggestions*

Living with Alzheimer's

Practical suggestions can aid in coping with the issues of everyday life with the Alzheimer's patient.

In the last chapter, we dealt with a few general principles regarding interactions between a caregiver and a person with Alzheimer's. In this chapter, we shall attempt to apply those principles to the practical situations of everyday life with an AD patient. As shown on the right, we first deal with issues concerning memory loss, especially focusing on communication skills. Then we discuss how those skills can be applied to designing safe living quarters, creating successful mealtimes and establishing a regular program of exercise and recreation. We then focus on personal hygiene issues, ranging from oral care and bathing to taking care of bodily wastes. Finally we discuss what to do in the advanced stages of Alzheimer's, and steps toward dealing with the finality of death.

You will notice that a common theme of this chapter is planning. In many cases, a crisis can be averted simply by preparing ahead of time for a particular situation. Because of Alzheimer's slow progression, there may be adequate time to, say, remodel a bathroom, create a list of people to call in a medical emergency, and so on. While every situation is different, the most practical suggestion of this chapter may also be the shortest: where possible, plan.

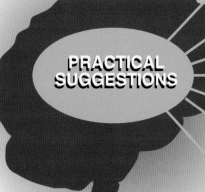

PRACTICAL
SUGGESTIONS

A FAMILIAR PERSPECTIVE

Throughout this chapter, we will deal with matters that most of us have always considered personal and private. We have been taught from a very early age to brush our own teeth, take our own baths and showers, display proper eating etiquette, go to the bathroom by ourselves. As the disease worsens, the Alzheimer's patient's ability to accomplish these same acts is hampered, and he will eventually need help, sometimes with even the simplest, most basic acts of living.

Assisting in such personal matters can be uncomfortable both for the person in charge *and* for the patient. It is important for caregivers to be able to discharge these feelings and work them out with other people in a non-stressful atmosphere. It is also important to remember that the person with AD may himself be ashamed and embarrassed at his deficits and lack of ability. As we have often discussed, it helps to acquire a certain amount of patience and perspective as a caregiver. Very few people would willingly embarrass, hurt or behave around caregivers the way a person with AD inadvertently might, because people without the disease have normal, unatrophied brains and nerve cells. The familiar refrain is: *Alzheimer's is a disease that the afflicted person cannot control.* It may be important to recall this as we discuss the practical issues in this chapter.

1 Memory loss

How to communicate with someone whose memory is failing. Dealing with clinging behaviors, sexual issues, etc.

2 Living quarters

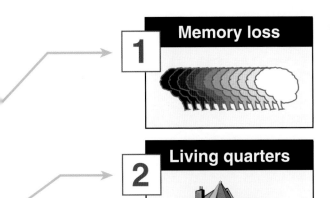

Making the living environment safe for someone progressively losing memory and coordination.

3 Mealtime

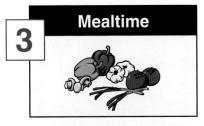

How to prepare meals, how to work with eating at mealtimes, coping with the loss of eating habits.

4 Exercise

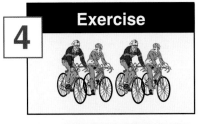

The importance of a regular exercise routine, how to make life more enjoyable for a person with AD.

5 Personal hygiene

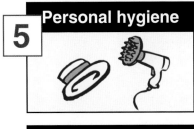

Grooming activities such as dressing, hair cutting, teeth brushing, bathing a person with Alzheimer's.

6 Bodily wastes

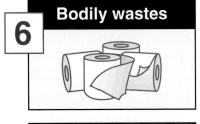

Dealing with urinary incontinence and fecal incontinence. How to design a bathroom for an AD patient.

7 At the end

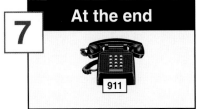

911

Making plans for long-term care and death. How to prepare for a medical crisis in the advanced stages of AD.

Verbal communication and memory loss with AD

The impact of Alzheimer's on memory can be easily observed in verbal communication. A caregiver must exercise a great deal of patience to communicate effectively.

We begin this chapter by suggesting ways to talk and listen to a person with Alzheimer's disease. As we have described earlier, memory loss can cause a person to forget the names of objects, of people, to endlessly ramble, to make grammatical mistakes when speaking, repeat the same thing over and over again, even misidentify common everyday objects. For example, Beth noticed that every time Daddy wanted to say the word "bacon," he said the word "freezer" instead. Researchers do not know exactly why this occurs, but it is helpful to think of Alzheimer's and verbal communication like a malfunctioning telephone system. Each time you pick up the phone to order pizza, you first get the police department, the next time the grocery store, the next time your next-door neighbor. Beth eventually learned that if she calmly asked Daddy a few questions, she could decipher what he was saying without risking a catastrophic reaction. And therein lies a key to learning to listen and speak to a person with AD. Listed below are some practical ways to communicate with an Alzheimer's patient.

Speaking to a person with Alzheimer's

ONE SUCCESSFUL APPROACH

The model that appears to have the greatest success in speaking to a person with AD has less to do with the words that are chosen (though these are important) than with the attitude behind the words. Caregivers who are unwavering in their responsiveness and consistently empathetic appear to communicate the most successfully. Put another way, people with Alzheimer's respond best to those who still treat them as adults, regardless of the disability.

One of the most difficult things to assess when speaking to a person with AD, however calm you are, is their comprehension. A person may hear the words, but interpret what is said very differently. It sometimes helps to reinforce your communication with nonverbal cues such as body language, pointing and gesturing, using facial expressions to make your verbal interactions more clear. The box on the right provides some suggestions that may help when verbal communication is required.

VERBALS IN SIX STEPS

#1) Address the person by his name.

#2) Pause a moment before continuing to make sure he is aware you are talking to him.

#3) Adjust the volume of your voice to his ability to hear you clearly.

#4) Speak briefly, using simple sentences and vocabulary.

#5) When finished speaking, pause again, allowing time for the patient to take in what you have said.

#6) Repeat steps 1-5 if necessary.

THE PROBLEM OF SILENCE

There may come a time when the patient simply stops talking. Whether he loses the meaning of so many words that verbal expression becomes impossible, or he just gives up due to the formidability of the effort, or none of these reasons, the patient lapses into silence. Losing verbal access to a patient can be a time of enormous difficulty for the caregiver, who must still respond and attend to the patient's needs.

Is there a solution? Nonverbal communication can help. Looking for cues in the patient such as eye movement, head nodding, angry pacing, even facial expressions, may communicate enough

information that the interpretation becomes clear. But not always; as we have discussed, some Alzheimer's behaviors have no reason outside of brain damage.

The caregiver can also use the same kinds of nonverbal communication to address the patient and provide reassurance, comfort, even direction. Touching, holding the patient's hand, exhibiting a calm countenance—these actions all say something potentially positive. Consistency in effort may be important as well, even if the results seem awkward at first, or at times even pointless.

Listening to a person with Alzheimer's

LISTENING AND CREATIVITY

The responsive empathy model for speaking works just as well for listening. It also helps to employ a little creativity, especially when the patient's verbals don't make sense. Consider the following conversation Beth taped one afternoon with her dad. They were talking about going to hear Beethoven's opera *Fidelio*.

DADDY: *You could bring the hot dogs to the auditorium.*

BETH: *Hot dogs? You don't bring hot dogs to an opera, Daddy. Why would you want hot dogs?*

DADDY: *Because somebody might give you the black tube things.*

BETH: *Black tube things? Do you mean socks?*

DADDY: *No. The black tube things. The ones with the string.*

BETH: *How about binoculars?*

DADDY: *Yeah, then you would have the binoculars.*

This example shows the creativity and patience a caregiver must sometimes employ to listen successfully to a patient with Alzheimer's. Beth did it without condescension, and in a way that kept her father from having a catastrophic reaction. Other practical suggestions are shown in the box on the right.

LISTENING IDEAS

#1) Supply the missing word when a person gets stuck. His frustration at not remembering the proper term may cause needless anger.

#2) Ask questions such as "How about ... ?" or "Do you mean ... ?" In the example on the right, Beth did this twice, once inquiring about socks, once asking about binoculars.

#3) Use nonverbal language to communicate consistent interest. If the person senses you are ignoring him, he may become angry, or worse, non-communicative.

Coping with other forms of memory loss in AD patients

The effects of memory loss can be seen in behaviors other than verbal communication. These include repetitive behaviors, inappropriate clinging, suspicion, depression, even rage.

Many human functions can be affected by memory loss, some of which are so subtle we don't realize that a problem is traceable to memory. Consider the perception of time, for example. Daddy once walked into a grocery store with Beth and, after five minutes, demanded to leave. When Beth asked him why, he said that they had been there for hours, he was beginning to feel abandoned, and he wanted to go home! To measure the passage of time we need memory, and when it fades, our ability to accurately assess the hours diminishes as well.

SEXUAL BEHAVIORS

Another subtle problem of memory is the perception of what constitutes socially acceptable behaviors. This is most often seen in issues of sexuality. In the support group Beth attended, a woman named Susan related that her father wanted to have sex with her and would yell out his feelings, calling out his wife's name, even in public. Not only was he confusing Susan with his wife, he had completely lost the memory of what was socially acceptable. Many patients disrobe in public and/or masturbate frequently and indiscreetly.

The issue with Susan's father had a happy ending. Beth suggested that he might really just be asking for physical comfort and reassurance through some kind of bodily contact. That turned out to be the case. Susan learned to hug her Dad more, and at various times during the day. That reduced the embarrassing behavior considerably.

Listed on this page are other behaviors that at first might not seem to be associated with memory loss, but very truly are. Where possible, suggestions are offered that may help caregivers to cope with what might seem baffling behavior. Since people experience Alzheimer's in different ways, these suggestions are only loose guidelines, and may or may not work in a given situation.

Behaviors that are

BEHAVIOR	DESCRIPTION
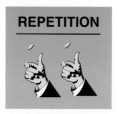 **REPETITION**	Patient repeats the same motion over and over again, sometimes for hours. The behavior may be verbal; patient makes the same statement or asks the same question incessantly.
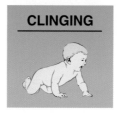 **CLINGING**	Caregiver is constantly shadowed by patient, to the point where personal habits are interrupted. Patient may become very anxious when caregiver goes out of sight.
 **SUSPICIONS**	Patient becomes suspicious beyond a reasonable level, overreacting even to neutral situations. Patient may accuse caregiver of stealing personal objects or of being part of a conspiracy.
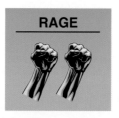 **RAGE**	Patient flies into uncontrollable anger. Can take many forms, including hitting, spitting, throwing objects, pinching. May become violent, threatening caregiver, others.

DEALING WITH DEPRESSION

Not surprisingly, people with Alzheimer's can suffer from clinical depression. In many cases, this occurs as the patient becomes increasingly aware of memory loss and debilitation. The great challenge for the caregiver is to discern which changes in behavior are associated with Alzheimer's and which are associated with depression. Since depression is a treatable illness, it is worthwhile to consult a medical professional as soon as it is suspected. Though they can be signs, not all depressions show symptoms of sadness and despondency. On the right is a checklist of symptoms that may indicate that a depression is present.

- Loss of energy, fatigue
- Listlessness, apathy
- Sudden hyperactivity
- Changes in appetite, digestive complaints
- Disturbances in sleeping patterns
- Sadness, feelings of despondency
- Suicidal tendencies
- Loss of interest in pleasurable activities and recreation
- Hypochondria

associated with memory loss and AD

WHAT TO DO

The origins of this behavior remain unknown. In at least some instances, the repetition is due to a disruption in short-term—and maybe even long-term—memory. Beth, for example, got extremely frustrated with her father when he asked her five times in a row what shirt he wore yesterday. Since clothes were very important to Daddy, Beth decided to make a list of the shirts and pants he was going to wear during the week. She then asked him to check it off every time he wore a particular article of clothing. This simple solution worked for a while, and instead of asking her repetitively, her father would pore over the list at various times throughout the week.

This kind of behavior may also be related to short- and long-term memory deficits. The patient may see the caregiver as a source of security, and may no longer realize that the caregiver does not disappear simply because she leaves the room. Beth's father never exhibited this behavior, but she did hear about examples from other caregivers in her support group. Some caregivers didn't seem to mind; their patients simply tagged along wherever the caregiver went. Other caregivers found that their patients could be distracted for periods of time by involving them in a project. That gave the caregiver time to attend to personal needs, such as taking a shower.

As objects begin to disappear from memory, a patient may try to organize the loss in as logical a fashion as possible. The person may conclude the objects were stolen, and perhaps, as possessions continue to be lost, that a conspiracy exists. Beth experienced this with Daddy in two ways. One was related to food (he thought he was being poisoned), the other with his bank account (he thought someone was stealing money). No matter what she tried, whether eating the food first in front of Daddy or showing him bank statements, nothing allayed his suspicions. What appeared to work best was creating distractions—asking Daddy to sweep the front porch, take a walk, play the piano, anything—when his accusations became strident. This solution actually worked for a long time.

Much of the time, rage reactions do not seem related to any discernible environmental cues or provocations on the part of the caregiver (and very often are quickly forgotten by the patient). In fact, no one really knows why these rages occur, and since the patient usually can't say why he is raging, little can be done in unprovoked attacks except to get out of the way. If the caregiver is the object of the anger and feels threatened, the caregiver must leave the situation immediately. Hospitals can be called (some even have Alzheimer's units) and an ambulance with personnel trained to handle the angry person can be sent to the home. The police can be notified as well, though in general, hospital personnel are better trained to handle such situations.

Securing the living quarters

The AD individual's living area can be filled with hazards, some obvious, some not. Here are a few suggestions about safeguarding.

Memory deficits do not just create the verbal and emotional communication problems described on the last few pages. Memory impairments also mean the person is increasingly less able to supervise his own personal safety. Because the brain damage is selective, it is not always easy to predict the issues that may be involved in safeguarding an AD patient. Since the damage increases over time, what works one month may not work the next. People who have cared for Alzheimer's patients have found practical ways to secure their living situations. They have found that the two most dangerous rooms in the house are the kitchen and the bathroom. Specific suggestions for securing these rooms, as well as general ideas for other parts of the living area, are listed here.

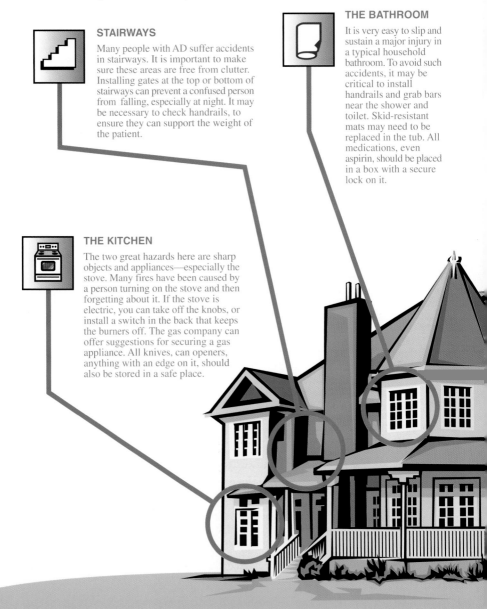

STAIRWAYS

Many people with AD suffer accidents in stairways. It is important to make sure these areas are free from clutter. Installing gates at the top or bottom of stairways can prevent a confused person from falling, especially at night. It may be necessary to check handrails, to ensure they can support the weight of the patient.

THE BATHROOM

It is very easy to slip and sustain a major injury in a typical household bathroom. To avoid such accidents, it may be critical to install handrails and grab bars near the shower and toilet. Skid-resistant mats may need to be replaced in the tub. All medications, even aspirin, should be placed in a box with a secure lock on it.

THE KITCHEN

The two great hazards here are sharp objects and appliances—especially the stove. Many fires have been caused by a person turning on the stove and then forgetting about it. If the stove is electric, you can take off the knobs, or install a switch in the back that keeps the burners off. The gas company can offer suggestions for securing a gas appliance. All knives, can openers, anything with an edge on it, should also be stored in a safe place.

Three general suggestions for modifiying the home

1   CLUTTER AND LIGHTING

A clean, well-lit house is always safer than a cluttered, poorly lit house. A person with AD may be inclined to trip over things more often in a cluttered house, especially in dim light (and even more, at night). A messy, dimly lit house is likely to cause an increase in the number of accidents.

2   HAZARDOUS MATERIALS

From power tools to insecticides, hazardous materials are perhaps the greatest single threat to an Alzheimer's patient. Guns, knives, hammers, nails, any potentially damaging hardware must always be stored in a locked, inaccessible storage area. Household cleaners, paints, solvents, pesticides can be placed in childproof cabinets, available at most hardware stores.

3   SUPERVISING SIMPLE TASKS

Guarding against accidents sometimes means supervising a person who is doing the everyday tasks of life. Alzheimer's disease is fully capable of disabling those parts of the brain responsible for remembering how to do simple things like using a can opener, cutting food. This loss can easily be overlooked by caregivers, resulting in unfortunate accidents.

FURNITURE

Furniture can be another source of injuries for AD patients. Items with sharp corners should be removed. Using stable, well-constructed chairs and removing ones that easily tip over (like rocking chairs) may help reduce accidents. Furniture upholstery should be treated so that it can be easily cleaned. Fabrics and curtains should be treated as well. The use of flame-resistant material whenever possible is recommended.

ADDING LOCKS

Installing security locks on doors and windows may be useful. Patients can sometimes lean too far out of windows and even balconies.

REMOVING LOCKS

People with AD can lock themselves into a room, with sometimes negative consequences. It may be beneficial to disable or even remove the locks from certain doors.

WATER HEATERS

People with AD can lose the ability to recognize that water is too hot; as a result, they often get burned. To prevent scalding, it may be important to lower the temperature on the water heater.

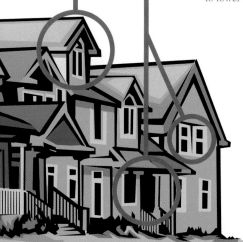

THE CAREGIVER REACTS

An unexpected source of accidents comes not from the patient, but from the caregiver. It has been shown that accidents are much more likely to occur in the home if the caregiver is angry or in a hurry. People tend to be less alert at these times and the rising tension can breed both carelessness and an adverse reaction in the patient. At these times, the best safety lesson is for the caregiver to slow down, taking time to release tension, changing the atmosphere to a more peaceful, relaxed state.

Dealing with mealtime: Part I

A challenging practical issue facing many caregivers of people with AD has to do with food preparation and consumption. The ideas presented in the next four pages seek to identify ways of working smoothly with Alzheimer's patients and their eating behaviors. We start by considering the following entry from Beth's journal, which in many ways typifies problems caregivers encounter at mealtime.

It seems like Daddy forgot that he just ate dinner! That's hysterical, because it sure was memorable for the rest of us. I had to lay an old tarp around his seat right in the middle of dinner because he started throwing his food on the floor. When that was done, he jumped out of his seat and dashed to his room with my sister in pursuit (she tried in vain to wash him up). Just as quickly he ran back—with Sis still following—and asked what was for dinner, because he said he was starving!

7/5/88

The problem with mealtime

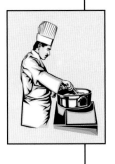

The simple act of eating regular meals can be traumatic for a person with Alzheimer's disease, and as Beth's journal highlights, for caregivers as well. The reason has to do with the number of sometimes-ritualized actions that must be remembered to consume food. In our culture, you feel the hunger, you remember that eating will satisfy the hunger, you sit at a table, you use certain utensils to put food on your plate, you use different utensils to take the food from the plate into your mouth, you chew your food, you swallow your food, then you use utensils to get more food.

Because AD destroys memory in a piecemeal fashion, part of the sequence may be remembered fully while other parts are completely forgotten. Shown below is the same sequence of events just described. The red text to the right describes what can happen to a person with the selective memory during mealtimes. On the next page are suggestions for dealing with the loss.

1

Feeling hunger.

Remembering that eating takes hunger away.

→ *A person with AD may not eat, even if food is in plain sight. This may occur for many reasons. For example, the person may not remember that eating can take the hunger away.*

2

Sitting at a table.

→ *A patient may not remember where food is served. He may not even remember how to sit in a chair when dinner is put on the table.*

3

Using kitchen utensils.

Placing food in the mouth.

→ *The memory of using a kitchen utensil may be lost. In some cases, the person can be retaught. In other cases, she may just stare at the food, not knowing how to get it into her mouth.*

4

Chewing the food.

Swallowing the food.

→ *A person with AD may remember how to get food in her mouth, but forget what to do once it is there. She may not remember to chew, or even to swallow. Even if the patient's memory is intact, brain damage may directly impair the ability to swallow.*

WHAT TO DO ABOUT HUNGER

People with Alzheimer's may not necessarily lose the memory of how to eat a meal, especially in the earlier stages of the disease. Rather, they may just begin to behave in an odd manner when they perceive their own hunger. A person with AD may, for example, begin to hoard, nibble or even eat inappropriate household items. Below is a description of these behaviors and suggestions about how to cope with them.

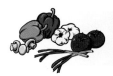

HOARDING

Some people will save food, hiding it in their rooms. A natural attractant to rodents and insects, this practice is a health risk.

Many patients will stop hoarding if they are reassured that they can have a snack any time they are hungry. Keeping a container filled with between-meal foods, and reminding the patient where it is, can provide such reassurance.

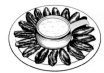

NIBBLING

Patients can forget they have already eaten, or simply develop a large appetite. They may seem to want to eat all the time.

The same solution as described above can work here—an open container of snacks available any time. If weight gain begins to be a problem, the snack container can be filled with things like carrots and celery.

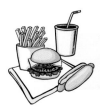

WRONG FOODS

Some people forget that some foods are bad for them. They may even eat non-food items, such as soap, dirt, and household plants.

This behavior may stem from brain damage in areas of perception as well as memory. The only solution is to remove the offending objects, keeping them out of sight and reach of the person with Alzheimer's.

What the caregiver can do

- Create regularly scheduled meals, whether hunger is indicated or not.
- Check for loose-fitting dentures, or other signs that eating may be an uncomfortable activity.
- Look for signs of depression, constipation, a small stroke.

- Seat the person at the table, in as comfortable and as natural a position as possible.
- Check to make sure that the person's physical needs, such as using the bathroom, have been taken care of before the meal begins.

- Model eating behavior, asking the person to imitate your actions.
- If the person cannot be retaught (Alzheimer's can permanently alter coordination skills), serve food that is easily manipulated with fingers.
- Place non-skid material under plates, bowls, making eating as easy as possible.

- Make foods that are easily swallowed, e.g., chopped meat, gelatins.
- Watch for choking; a person with difficulty swallowing may choke or gag on food or pills. It may be useful to grind up pills and place into easily swallowed food. Becoming familiar with the Heimlich maneuver is important in caring for a swallowing-impaired person.

Dealing with mealtime: Part II

It is important, then, to remember that an AD patient may forget some of the basic eating functions taught in childhood. It is also important to remember that this memory loss may be selective, and while the patient may lose some abilities, other actions can be carried out normally. Part of making mealtime run more smoothly is to recognize which functions are present and which are not.

While keeping the memory loss in mind, another significant way to make mealtimes more stable has to do with creating a calming environment, one that will not lead to catastrophic reactions. These two pages outline ways such security may be achieved, and the active role a caregiver can play in making the preparation and consumption of food as successful as the disease will allow.

PREPARING FOOD

There is no special diet that will help alleviate the symptoms of Alzheimer's, and indeed none that can improve memory even in a healthy person. But following the common rules of good nutrition is as important to a person with AD as it is to anyone else—deficiencies in the diet will hurt a patient's function as surely as it would hurt the caregiver's. There are two ideas which may be helpful to remember in preparing foods for Alzheimer's patients.

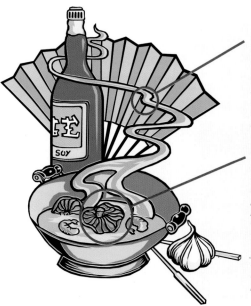

TEMPERATURE
People with Alzheimer's disease can lose the ability to judge the harmfulness of all kinds of environmental inputs, including the hot and cold sensations of food. It may become important to check the temperature of foods before they are served, especially if the food has been heated in a microwave oven.

FAMILIARITY
Some patients develop rigid standards of what they will and will not eat at mealtime (though if they did not like a particular food before the disease, they probably won't like it now). New foods may be confusing. Cooking familiar meals and preparing them in familiar ways can sometimes reduce the finickiness. A doctor may need to be consulted about vitamins and supplements if efforts at persuading a person to eat a balanced meal fail.

DEALING WITH MESSINESS

When fingers, hands and brain no longer work in a cooperative fashion, inevitable spills and messes result. In reaction, the patient may resort to using his fingers instead of the kitchen utensils on the table. He may no longer be able to drink from a normal cup. These behaviors are an inevitable consequence of AD's march across the human brain; it is usually much better to accommodate than to fight. Meals may need to be served in an area that is easily cleaned. A tarp or plastic tablecloth may be used on the floor, and a bib may need to be placed, with permission, on the patient. Scoop plates (or plate guards) can be bought from medical supply houses. The use of heavy dishes, or anti-slip devices placed under the dish (even a wet cloth), may help prevent slippage. It is possible to purchase spill-proof containers, such as convalescent feeding cups or cups made for toddlers for fluids served at the table.

AT THE TABLE

As mentioned, one of the most important ways to maintain a smoothly running meal has to do with creating an unconfusing, stable atmosphere at the table. This may not be as easily accomplished as one might think, since different patients can be confused about different things at mealtimes. Listed below are a few suggestions that may help create a calming, non-distracting environment for a person with AD.

A person with AD may get confused by the presence of salt and pepper shakers (or even other condiment holders, like a sugar bowl). It may be best to put these out of sight during the meal.

Use a plate that contrasts with the table or placemat (a white dish on a blue tablecloth, for example).

To a person with Alzheimer's, an array of kitchen utensils can be confusing. It may be helpful to put out only one utensil, like a fork, for the duration of the meal.

Putting several foods onto a plate all at once may bewilder a person with AD. It may be helpful to serve him foods consecutively, one at a time, during the meal.

Some foods may be difficult to cut into bite-sized pieces. The caregiver may need to cut certain foods, like meat, before serving.

So that the person with AD can see the plate, the food, and utensils plainly, it may be necessary to add additional lighting to the dining area.

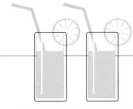

KEEPING UP WITH FLUIDS

Even people in the initial stages of AD often forget to drink enough fluids (that goes for most of us, in fact, whether we suffer from Alzheimer's or not). Not drinking enough fluids can lead to physical problems listed on the right. It is important that the caregiver pay attention to the amount of fluids being taken by the patient. This becomes especially critical if the patient has been vomiting or suffering from diarrhea, is diabetic, or is taking certain kinds of heart medication.

SYMPTOMS OF DEHYDRATION

- Thirst
- Refusal to drink fluids
- Fever
- Flushing (turning red)
- Pale lining in the mouth
- Rapid pulse
- Dizziness, lightheadedness
- Hallucinations
- No urine output

Personal hygiene: Part I

The amount of personal hygiene care a patient with Alzheimer's needs varies with the amount of brain damage. As time progresses, assistance with personal issues such as dressing and grooming may be required.

As Alzheimer's destroys progressively more regions of the brain, the person with AD is less and less able to fend for herself. In the beginning stages of the disease, she can usually fulfill most of her own personal hygiene needs. But personal behaviors, such as dressing and grooming, get more difficult as her memory begins to fade.

Dealing with personal hygiene isssues can be extremely difficult, both for the patient and the caregiver. There are two reasons for this. First, we are all used to doing our personal functions in a certain way, and usually without an audience. Many of us, in fact, have never bathed or dressed in front of anyone on a routine basis. In the next four pages, we will address the topics of dressing, grooming, bathing, and oral hygiene. These two ideas, that people have their own ways of performing personal routines, and that we usually do them in private, must be considered.

DRESSING A PERSON WITH ALZHEIMER'S

Getting dressed involves many complex choices as well as specific memory skills. These tasks can sometimes be overwhelming to a person with Alzheimer's disease. Here are some suggestions that may help eliminate some of the confusion:

We are finally getting the routine down, but I have to stay with Daddy to make sure he does it right. It's his clothes routine. If I don't stuff his pajamas into the dresser the instant he takes them off, he very quickly puts them on again. Then I have to make sure he puts his underwear on before his pants, or he gets all confused and starts throwing his briefs around the room. Lately, he's been putting his pants on backwards, and then starts doing this weird dance, like he's trying to screw his pants around so that the zipper will be in the front like normal. At first I didn't know what he was doing. But after a bit, I understood, and after some arguments and hassle, he let me put them on right for him. Thank God that's the only time this is difficult. If he gets it all right, with his clothes put on in the right order, he'll stay dressed all day.

• Lay out in advance an entire outfit for the person to wear. The clothing can even be placed on a bed in the order they are to be put on.

• Throw out or put into storage clothing that is either seldom or never worn. Reducing the number of choices a patient must make can make the task of dressing much smoother.

• Eliminate unneeded accessories. Scarves, sweaters, belts, items of jewelry, and so on can sometimes make choices for apparel unnecessarily complex even in undiseased people. Simplifying a patient's choices, as stated above, can provide a calming influence.

• Simplify the way things are put on. Zippers, buttons, and ties can be difficult to use for a confused person who is also losing her coordination. Replacing such items with Velcro fasteners, or buying clothing that needs only to be slipped on (such as T-shirts, sweats, and shoes that do not need to be tied) can reduce stress both for the caregiver and the patient. Loose-fitting clothing is easier to work with as well.

• Select clothing that is simple to manage. It may be best to buy apparel that needs little ironing and can hold up well to repeated washing. Apparel with colors that provide high-contrast can be more easily distinguished by a person with AD. Conversely, clothing with complex patterns can confuse and distract the patient. Selections that can easily mix-and-match with each other do not depend upon "proper" decisions in order to look attractive and natural.

As caregivers, it is important to remember that people with Alzheimer's can be very aware that something is wrong. The physical deterioration of their bodies can greatly add to their confusion, even if they do not always understand perfectly what is happening. As personal hygiene issues are addressed, it is important to keep in mind that the patient is still an adult, and may have normal reactive feelings (such as fear, confusion, and humiliation) to their sudden need for intimate help. This confusion, can be greatly aggravated by decreased physical ability.

Mental confusion can be aggravated by decreased physical ability

GROOMING A PERSON WITH ALZHEIMER'S

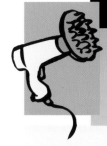

Personal grooming skills, such as getting haircuts and shaving, can be increasingly forgotten by people with AD. Since they also involve a sequence of memorized events, personal grooming tasks can be as confusing to an Alzheimer's patient as dressing. Below are suggestions for how to make personal grooming less difficult.

My brother's girlfriend hit on a great idea. I had been having trouble getting Daddy to shave for a couple of weeks, and his face was starting to look just awful. She asked me if Daddy ever went to a barber—and that maybe Daddy got a shave after he got a haircut. I told her no, but then I wasn't sure. So I called the barber, and asked him if he remembered Daddy. Then I asked him if he would be willing to come over and give him a shave, maybe even a haircut at the same time. He said yes, he remembered Daddy just fine, and would come over after work. What do you know? Daddy not only allowed him to shave, but also allowed him to cut his hair. I have decided to set this up on a regular basis.

• Determine whether a barber or beautician is really needed. People who have gone to a hair professional all their lives may wish to continue doing so. But if such trips become too confusing, it may be possible for the caregiver to arrange for the professional to come to the home (see Beth's entry on the left).

• Simplify the patient's hairstyle. It may eventually be important to cut the hair of a person with AD in a short, attractive style that is easy to wash and maintain. Avoid a style that requires setting.

• Create a place where the patient's hair is easily washed. It is generally easier on the caregiver's back, and safer all around, if hair is washed in a sink rather than in a tub. It may be important to buy a hose attachment to a deep sink, such as in a kitchen, to create a place where hair is washed conveniently.

• Attention to trimming fingernails and toenails is important. It can sometimes be easy to forget such details, having assumed a patient might do this for themselves under normal circumstances. But even the pain and discomfort of ingrown nails can go untreated if the patient has forgotten how to use proper clipping utensils, or does not identify the reason for the pain.

• If the patient is a male, there may come a time when the caregiver will need to learn to shave his face. This can be difficult for both parties. The solution Beth employed with her barber may work for some patients. Regardless of the solution, it is always safer to use an electric razor than a manual razor.

• It is possible that the patient, especially if female, may try to put on makeup and fail; the caregiver may need to learn to apply it for her (though some professionals suggest to avoid makeup if at all possible, especially eye makeup). If the patient insists on wearing it, the task may be simplified. A simple application of powder and lipstick may suffice.

Personal hygiene: Part II

Here we explore issues of cleaning, bathing, and oral hygiene.

BATHING A PERSON WITH ALZHEIMER'S

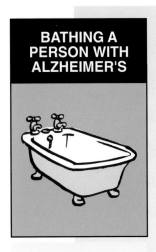

Bathing can sometimes be a difficult task for a caregiver and the patient. Sometimes the person with Alzheimer's does not feel he needs a bath, even if he has begun to smell bad. Sometimes a patient seems to develop a genuine fear of a shower. The negative reaction may include the perception that the task is too overwhelming, too complicated, too confusing. These responses can be very frustrating for a caregiver, especially because it is critical, for health reasons, that some kind of bathing ritual be established. Listed here are some suggestions that may help bathing a person with AD to go more smoothly.

There are times when the only thing I can do is laugh. This morning I tried to give Daddy a bath, like I always do. But this time he kept refusing, saying that he didn't need a bath. So I kept it up. I told him to take the washcloth I was holding—which he did—and then I told him to unbutton his pajamas. Once again he said that he didn't need to take a bath, and at the same time, he started fumbling around with his pajama tops. Eventually he got his clothes off, all the time telling me he wasn't going to take a bath. So finally I told him to step into the water. And he did, still insisting he wasn't going to take a bath. I told him fine, and then I almost laughed out loud!

• Establish a ritual. Bathtime should consist of a regular, predictable routine. Since feelings of security are large issues for many AD patients, doing the bath the same way at the same time may make him come to expect it and hence, put up less resistance. It may not be necessary to bathe the person every day.

• Follow closely his original bathing habits. Many patients become more cooperative if an attempt is made to do things in a manner similar to their pre-disease routine. For example, if the person always showered in the morning, then shaved, then went down to breakfast, it may be useful for the caregiver to follow that same order when establishing a bathing routine.

• Be creative, rather than forcefully aggressive, in getting the patient to bathe. Gentle manipulation can sometimes go a lot further than screaming and yelling. For example, the caregiver may put water into a bathtub beforehand, then show the patient the water, entreating him to take a bath since "the water is already there." It may help to avoid getting into discussions about whether to take a bath, but instead gently persist, as shown in Beth's example on the left.

• Watch the water temperature. People with Alzheimer's disease can lose the ability to perceive the correct water temperature. This loss can be quite sudden, leading to scalding or an uncomfortably cold bathing experience. The temperature should always be tepid, and tested by the caregiver before the bath. You don't always need to fill the tub with water; sometimes only two or three inches will suffice.

• Be careful in getting a person in and out of the tub. Slippery water and soap are tricky for people without coordination problems; with Alzheimer's, such situations can be disastrous for both patient and caregiver. Installing handrails may be useful. New bathmats may be essential. It is possible to buy or rent a "bath seat" and a handheld hose, where the patient is seated in the bathtub and "showered" by the caregiver using the hose. Sometimes a sponge bath is the only kind of bathing a patient can handle.

• Be thorough in your cleansing and drying. Be sure to wash the patient's genitals, since harmful infections may develop if the area is not thoroughly cleansed. Make sure after the bath that the person is completely dried off. Body powders, even baking soda can be used as effective body deodorants. Drying time can be an opportune moment to check for red spots (a first sign of so-called bedsores), rashes or other skin irritations.

The resistance patients can display regarding personal hygiene activities such as bathing and brushing teeth can be intense. It may help caregivers to remember that this is a normal human reaction, that they too might react in a similar fashion if someone tried to interfere with the private details of their lives. A person with AD may forget how to brush his teeth, yet still retain adult behaviors and memories for many other tasks of daily life. As we have often said, Alzheimer's involves a loss of brain cells, but can be very selective in the memories it destroys.

ORAL HYGIENE AND ALZHEIMER'S

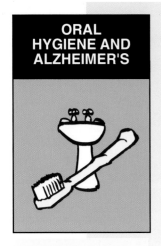

Once again Daddy has refused to eat. He keeps telling me that he's not hungry, and I know that it can't be true. He only had some juice since last evening. And his breath smelled so bad this afternoon that I thought something was rotting! So I took Daddy to the dentist, and the dentist immediately found what was wrong. He said it looked like Daddy hadn't cleaned his false teeth in a long time, and that the rotten smell was part food and part infection. Then the dentist asked me if Daddy has been eating lately, and I was shocked that he would ask that question. But he said something really interesting. The dentist told me that some people quit eating when their mouth hurts too much, and that he thinks Daddy's mouth really hurts. He gave me some medicine and mouthwashes, which he said should help.

Another task that can be difficult for both caregiver and patient involves maintaining oral hygiene. It can be especially easy to overlook simply because problems can lie hidden for so long. And a patient who can still take care of himself in other ways may simultaneously be forgetting dental hygiene. As ever, the biggest problem is that brushing one's teeth is not a simple procedure, but rather involves a series of complex tasks given in a specific sequence. A person may lose the memory of part but not all of the routine, which can create difficulties between him and his caregiver. Listed here are some suggestions that may help.

• Let the person do as much of the task as possible. Once again, most people are used to doing the personal tasks of everyday life in a specific, private way. Allowing the person as much freedom to brush his teeth or clean his dentures as he sees fit is a paramount goal. From the caregiver's point of view, the most important objective is that proper hygiene occurs.

• Establish a regular routine. The mechanics of oral hygiene may be resisted less if the patient knows it is a part of an expected, regular routine. The caregiver may need to choose a time of the day when the person is least resistant to suggestions and input. If the patient gets upset, it may be important to try again another time.

• When difficulties occur, break tasks down into easily understood, individual tasks. When the patient has difficulties with brushing his teeth or cleaning his dentures, it may be important to discover what part of the sequence is being forgotten. This can be discovered by separating the process of brushing and cleaning into discrete steps.

• Learn proper brushing technique. There may come a time when the caregiver has to take over most of the oral hygiene chores. It may be wise to consult with a dentist to learn how to do this properly. Some patients may resist such intimate interference, putting up a fight and clenching their teeth. Patience and gentleness are the most important attitudes for a caregiver during such times; even clenched teeth can be cleaned from the outside. Some dentists recommend foam applicators over brushes. Others recommend glycerine peroxide solutions or even mouthwashes (it is important that the patient be instructed not to swallow these, and he may need to be taught to spit out the liquid).

• If the person with AD has dentures, these must be cleaned and must adhere properly. Examine the fit of the patient's dentures, asking him if his teeth hurt, looking for abnormal mouth movement. Many patients stop eating if chewing becomes painful. This can lead to malnutrition and a host of associated problems. To maximize chewing comfort, it is important that the caregiver sees that the dentures fit and that they are being attached properly.

• If proper cleaning of dentures is neglected, painful sores on the gum can develop. This interferes with the ability to chew, of course, and hence with proper nutrition. If the caregiver becomes responsible for denture maintenance, they must be cleaned once a day and the gums checked for irritation. A dentist can show the caregiver the proper procedures for cleaning dental appliances.

Dealing with urinary incontinence and Alzheimer's

"It was easily my worst nightmare, though I knew the day would eventually come. Daddy peed in his pants for the first time today. I was so upset—and grossed out— that I cried and cried. But I just couldn't let him walk around smelling like pee all day, and Rachel told me the wetness would be bad for his skin. I finally got the nerve to change his clothes. And then I spent the rest of the day in the garden."

One of the most unfortunate consequences of Alzheimer's disease is that people like Daddy may start to lose control over the bladder and bowel functions. Called respectively urinary and fecal incontinence, these twin problems are usually unrelated. They will be dealt with separately in the next four pages, beginning with urinary incontinence.

We have been taught since we were little that getting rid of bodily wastes is a private function. It is a symbol of our independence and dignity as human beings that we be able to do such tasks on our own. When such powerful social forces no longer hold sway over a patient, a caregiver must begin to assess why the change has occurred. In the case of urinary continence, a number of important questions must be asked, some of which are shown below.

Do accidents happen only at night? At other times of the day?

If the patient is female, is she leaking, rather than completely emptying her bladder?

How often does the person go to the bathroom?

Is the urination painful?

Do accidents happen only once in a while? Regularly?

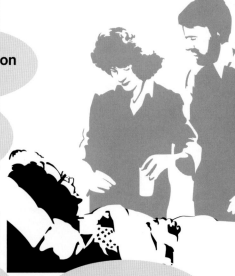

Do the accidents happen on the way to the bathroom?

Is the patient living in a new room? New place?

Does the patient urinate in some place other than the toilet?

There are many reasons urinary incontinence occurs. Regardless of the problem, the first thing the caregiver must rule out when confronting the "accidents" is a medical condition. Incontinence can occur because of bladder infections, diabetes, dehydration, medications, even an enlarged prostate. As we discussed in an earlier chapter, leaking can occur because of weakening muscles. A trip to the doctor can help determine if such conditions are present. Many times, medically related conditions can be treated.

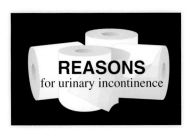

REASONS
for urinary incontinence

Once a medical reason has been ruled out, a caregiver must look for other problems that lead to accidents. For example, a person may just move too slowly to get to the bathroom on time. Or she may lose the ability to undo a zipper or a button in a hurry. A patient may not be able to find the bathroom, especially if she is in a new living environment (or she may forget where the bathroom is, even if she has lived in the same house for many years). Of course the amount of fluid intake is important. Surprisingly, incontinence can occur if the person is getting too *little* fluid. A certain amount is needed to stimulate the bladder to work, which means that incontinence can occur if the person is getting too much *or* too little fluid throughout the day.

SOME PRACTICAL SUGGESTIONS

Beth was very unsure about what to do with Daddy's "problem." The doctor told her that nothing was physically wrong that he could treat, and so Beth was left to figure out the situation on her own. The first thing she did was to fit all the furniture in the house with washable seat covers. Then, acting on Rachel's advice, she started making a diary of when Daddy usually went to the bathroom. That gave her some clues as to possible "emergency" times, when he was most likely to have an accident. Shown below are entries describing some of the other things she tried in an effort to cope with her father's incontinence.

Daddy started to wet his pants fairly constantly at night. I thought maybe that he couldn't find his way to the bathroom, so I put up some nightlights in the hall. I even put up a big sign that said "Bathroom" in big red letters with an arrow. Then I started worrying about him tripping and falling, so Rachel suggested that I put a mini-toilet in his room, like the ones you find in hospitals. That seemed to work for awhile.

I finally took all of Daddy's pants and ripped out the zippers. The poor guy was all over himself trying to unzip his jeans so he could pee. I could even tell he had to go, because he tried to unzip his pants in front of the living room vase (he has actually peed there before!). Anyway, I replaced the zippers with Velcro and now he doesn't have to fumble around, though sometimes he just stands at the toilet, like he's wanting to use it.

I think I got this peeing stuff down now, without having to buy those adult diaper things. I found that if I woke Daddy up around 2:30 every morning and had him go to the bathroom, he could make it through the night without wetting the bed. In the daytime, I have started to to take him to the toilet every three hours or so, even if he doesn't seem like he needs to pee. He hasn't had an accident in almost three days!

Dealing with fecal incontinence and Alzheimer's

As described on the previous page, fecal incontinence is the inability of a person to control bowel movements. Just like urinary incontinence, such difficulties may be an indication of a medical problem. These can include infection, diarrhea, constipation, or a condition known as fecal impaction (the intestine becomes completely blocked). It is important to have a doctor examine the patient; in some cases, fecal incontinence can be treated.

It is also important to remember that fecal incontinence is not necessarily related to its urinary counterpart. A person may control his bladder easily, and still have problems soiling his pants (or vice versa). In the diary entry below, Beth discovered that Daddy was able to control his bowel movements long after he had lost control of his bladder.

The other shoe finally dropped this morning. I had thought it would take a lot less time than this, but for the first time, Daddy messed his pants. God knows Daddy had been wetting his pants for many months, and I thought this would come right along with it. It was really odd, and maybe there's a hint in this. Daddy spent about an hour in the bathroom this morning, sitting on the toilet and just kind of staring into space.

I called that dear Rachel, and she told me to visit the doctor (what a surprise). The doctor told me that I might want to make our bathroom a little more friendly for Daddy, especially if this problem continues. I thought I would be a lot more disgusted with this than I am, especially because the bathroom will cost money. Maybe it's from cleaning up after Daddy's peeing. Maybe it's the look on Daddy's face when I clean him up. He doesn't seem to be putting up much of a fight these days. Now he just seems extremely sad. Mom said he actually helped change all the kids' diapers when we were little. I wonder if I will have to return the favor.

Support devices may need to be professionally installed. The patient should have something to hold onto. This will not only aid the person getting on and off the seat, but may encourage a restless person to stay put.

TOILET DESIGN

Beth eventually heard from her doctor and found, as with the urinary problem, there was nothing medically wrong. Several things were done to the toilet Daddy frequented that made it easier to use. The kinds of adjustments made are shown on the drawing. The doctor told Beth to keep, as unobtrusively as possible, records of her father's bowel movements, even as she had made a diary about his urinary habits. Beth found that Daddy consistently moved his bowels about the same time every day, and as with the urination, began taking Daddy to the bathroom at that time of day, whether he felt like he needed to go or not. This worked only sometimes, and Beth eventually began to contemplate using adult diapers.

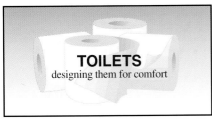

TOILETS
designing them for comfort

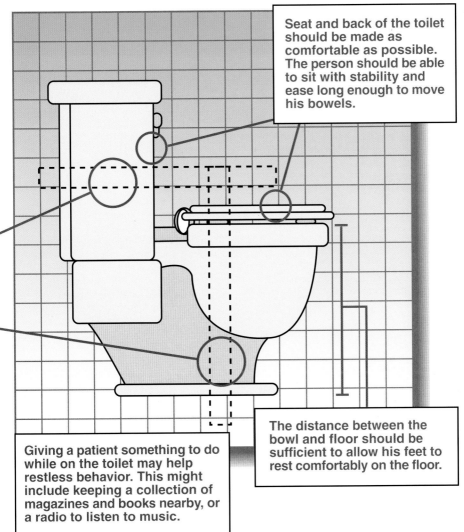

Seat and back of the toilet should be made as comfortable as possible. The person should be able to sit with stability and ease long enough to move his bowels.

The distance between the bowl and floor should be sufficient to allow his feet to rest comfortably on the floor.

Giving a patient something to do while on the toilet may help restless behavior. This might include keeping a collection of magazines and books nearby, or a radio to listen to music.

ARE DIAPERS APPROPRIATE?

It is easy for caregivers to become weary of cleaning up after incontinent patients. Professionals disagree if adult "diapers" are appropriate alternatives for people who have trouble controlling bodily excretions, however. Some feel that such apparel is potentially very discouraging to a patient, and may even encourage childlike responses and behaviors. Others believe that scheduling regular bathroom breaks is more effective and easier than wearing and changing diapers. Fortunately, there is no hard and fast rule, regardless of what a caregiver may hear. The solution lies solely in the feelings of the caregiver and the reactions of the patient. Employing diapers may make household life more convenient. Moreover, the patient may feel more secure wearing something than constantly worrying about his bowel and bladder functions.

Exercise and recreation

Proper exercise and recreation are as important to a person with AD as they are to anyone else. Here are some ways to keep an Alzheimer's patient active.

As you have heard many times, it is very important to establish and maintain a regular routine of physical and recreational activity. Such liveliness serves the additional role of stress reduction in the mental health of AD patients and their caregivers. Here are a few suggestions for physical activity and recreation that caregivers may consider as they interact with their patients.

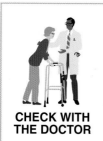

CHECK WITH THE DOCTOR

In planning exercise for a person with AD, the most important first activity may be to check with the person's physician. If the patient has complicating medical conditions, such as heart problems or high blood pressure, certain activities may be off-limits. The medical professional may also offer advice on how to start slowly and gradually build to a rigorous exercise program.

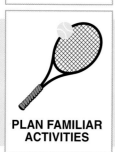

PLAN FAMILIAR ACTIVITIES

After determining the physical limits, the next set of decisions involves choosing the right activities. Important clues can come from the patient's past. If he liked a certain form of exercise prior to disease onset, such as dancing, he may still very much enjoy moving to music. Additionally, many people with AD enjoy doing calisthenics in a group setting. Exercises can even be done if the patient is bedridden.

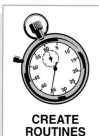

CREATE ROUTINES

Establishing a regular routine is as important for exercising as it is for the other aspects of an AD patient's life. The physical activities should take place at the same time every day, for example. The routines should be simple and presented in such a fashion as to avoid catastrophic reactions. With a little creativity, the physical activity can be made enjoyable, even fun, something to which the patient looks forward.

RECREATION

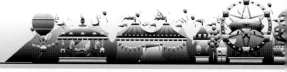

A diagnosis of Alzheimer's does not mean an end to enjoying life. But the caregiver may need to be creative in planning pleasurable activities appropriate to the severity of the disability (people with AD often lose the ability to entertain themselves). Like exercise, the caregiver may need to discern what activities the patient enjoyed prior to the illness, and then be imaginative in implementing specific activities. Many patients enjoy seeing old friends. Music can be an enjoyable experience, either listening to or singing familiar songs. Adult day-care programs can be a source of recreation, providing fellowship and camaraderie with other AD patients; well-structured programs can mix an appropriate amount of stimulation within a secure environment. Consider what happened to Beth's father one afternoon at a day care center in which Beth had enrolled him.

FRINGE BENEFITS

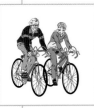

Medical professionals who work with AD patients have observed that exercise can sometimes improve certain behaviors. It has been shown, for example, that regular exercise can reduce the amount of agitated pacing an Alzheimer's patient may do, and may even make him calmer throughout the day. Physical activity can help a patient sleep better at night, can even help keep bowel movements on a regular schedule. Even though some people experience these "fringe benefits," it is important to remember that AD is not caused because of a lack of exercise, or from improper circulation, or any other condition that exercise may alleviate in a normal person.

5/24/90

For the second time this month I got chewed out by Daddy's doctor. It's not like I haven't tried to get Daddy to go out on walks with me. Maybe the doctor wants to get rid of Daddy's stiff joints by offering to go jogging with him instead of ME. Anyway, he had the gall to suggest I had to make Daddy more active, or face the fact that he'll get weaker and then get tired more easily. I said that I would.

5/25/90

I took out Daddy's old tennis racket from the attic. It was in pretty bad shape, and I didn't know how to get it restrung, but that didn't seem to matter. As soon as Daddy saw the racket, his eyes got very bright. He grabbed the racket and started making swooshing noises. I thought maybe we could hit some balls together outside against the garage wall. Maybe that will get him out of the house more.

5/26/90

The tennis "game" was a GREAT success! I actually enjoyed playing with Daddy, and he seemed happy to be doing it with me. It's not even close to being a real match; I just throw the ball to him and he tries to hit it against the wall. But I haven't seen him this enthusiastic to get out of the house in a long time. In fact, we have started doing it first thing every morning, when he has a lot of energy, just after he does his bathroom stuff.

So Daddy has become a concert piano player! Today at day care he fooled just about everybody. He isn't normally the center of attention, though he appears to really love going. He especially likes playing the piano in the back room. Today, one of the new attendants heard him playing and got an idea. She placed a bunch of chairs around the piano while Daddy was playing, and then asked some of the residents to come in, sit, and listen. To our complete surprise, Daddy looked up, saw all the people, burst into a great big smile and gave a small concert, playing for about half an hour! The attendant said he should do this regularly, and Daddy was in such a good mood when he got home that I agreed.

Planning for the end

The issues that surround the end stages of Alzheimer's disease are varied and complex. These involve choosing care facilities as well as attending to legal and medical issues.

The caregiver who is in charge of the life of a person with AD must also face the certainty of the patient's complete debilitation and, finally, death. It is much easier to deal with such a difficult time if a number of practical questions are settled prior to the debilitation. Important issues include preparing for advanced illness, as well as confronting certain legal and medical decisions. Some of these issues are described below.

ADVANCED CARE

There may come a time when the caregiver feels she can no longer take care of the patient. Twenty-four-hour care is exhausting for anyone, and many people are relieved to let professionals provide for the final months, even years, of an Alzheimer's patient's life.

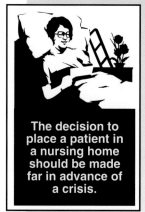

The decision to place a patient in a nursing home should be made far in advance of a crisis.

Ideally, the decision to place a patient in a nursing home should be made far in advance of a crisis situation. There are several reasons for this. First, finding the right long-term care facility can be a lengthy, arduous task. Everyone has heard the horror stories, and while most "snake pits" have long since been put out of business, not all facilities are perfect for every situation. Selection takes time, and getting into the best facilities usually requires a waiting list. Second, working in advance allows the patient to participate in the selection process. Allowing him to ask questions and getting his input as to preferences can be helpful in the painful decisions that must be made later on, especially when the patient may not be able to voice his opinion. Third, creating time to plan allows varying opinions of family members and/or friends to be aired without the added pressure of time. Consider this entry in Beth's journal regarding a family meeting about her father, a meeting that occurred several years before Daddy died.

7/25/88

After almost two months of dinners, I think the fighting is just about over. In my heart of hearts, I know Bill was right. Though I would never admit it, the hostility was mostly on my part. I just couldn't see Daddy sitting around in a bed being taken care of by someone young enough to be his grandson. I don't know why Bill's nose was bent out of joint anyway. It was *me* who volunteered to take Daddy in, for God's sake. Fortunately for us—especially after this last meeting—it all seemed to be a good compromise. If Sis helps him out, Bill will probably do a good job of getting Daddy on some waiting list for the best nursing home, and by the time we're ready, I'll probably be too burnt out to put up much of a fight anyway.

LEGAL PREPARATION

Aside long-term care, a difficult issue for caregivers is determining when the patient has reached the final stages of the disease. It is equally hard to know exactly how long the "final stages" will continue until death occurs (the body can stay alive for years after the brain ceases to provide adequate function). That's why it is important to obtain competent professional legal advice as soon as possible, helping to prepare the affairs of the patient far in advance of the end stages. Once again, early preparation will allow time for the caregivers to solicit the wishes of the patient. There is no one plan that will work for every family, of course. And since laws vary from state to state, some form of expert guidance is usually required. A few of the most important legal issues to consider are shown below.

DURABLE POWER OF ATTORNEY	LIVING TRUST	STANDARD WILL
Or DPA, this is a document allowing one individual to designate another person to act legally on the individual's behalf.	A living trust allows a person, while still alive, to designate someone else to manage some or all of the person's assets according to specific terms.	This is a document dictating how the assets belonging to a person's estate will be distributed upon the death of the person.

LIVING WILL	CONSERVATORSHIP OF PROPERTY	GUARDIANSHIP OF PERSON
This is an overall term for a document specifying the kinds of medical decisions to be made if the person loses mental competence.	A person may be designated by a court to manage assets of another individual if that individual is incapable of managing her estate.	A guardian may be appointed by a court if a patient becomes unable to care for his personal needs. Though available, this instrument is seldom used.

OTHER LEGAL MATTERS

In addition to the concerns listed above, it may be important for caregivers to a) review the nature of the ownership of the patient's property, b) remember to file tax returns for the patient (by durable power of attorney), c) review entitlements for which the person may be eligible. Entitlements are financial support devices such as Social Security Disability, Medicare and Medicaid.

MEDICAL PREPARATION

In the end stages of the disease, the last set of issues that must be addressed are the medical ones. Perhaps the most difficult of all, these issues revolve around how to deal with cessation of treatment and dying. People who have gone through the experience say that unless some advanced, explicit instructions are posted, surviving loved ones exercise startlingly little control over what occurs. Listed below are questions caregivers should consider as they prepare for the ending stages of the disease.

• What kind of medical intervention should be done if the patient becomes very ill? What about feeding tubes? What about antibiotic treatment or surgery for nonrelated concurrent illnesses? Much of this can be dealt with via the Living Will.

• If the person is in a nursing home, what is the institution's policy regarding medical intervention? Will resuscitation be attempted in case of an emergency? Will an ambulance be called? Can written instructions concerning intervention be placed in the patient's chart? Make sure the physician is aware of how these issues have been decided.

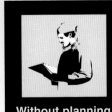

Without planning, surviving family members may exercise little control over what occurs with their loved ones.

There are very few "better" or "worse" choices when it comes to answering these questions. Indeed, clergy, lawyers, and medical professionals still wrestle with such issues without coming to much consensus. Whatever the decision, it is most important that the patient receive gentle care and be kept as pain-free as modern medicine will allow.

When death comes

Planning is an essential component of preparing for the death of someone with Alzheimer's. Here are some issues to consider.

In Chapter Two, we discussed how death occurs in Alzheimer's disease. The damage becomes so great on the patient's nervous system that the rest of the body is permanently affected. Eventually, vital functions begin to fail and the person's body, unable to cope with the ravages of the disease, dies. The immediate cause of death is often some kind of complicating illness, such as infection, pneumonia, or dehydration. But the actual cause of death is Alzheimer's disease.

Many people with Alzheimer's disease, like Beth's father, die in some kind of long-term care facility. Loved ones are often notified of death through a phone call. Other patients die at home, a fact that can cause a great deal of anxiety on the part of some caregivers. They can become afraid to sleep deeply; they might even find themselves getting up several times a night just to check on the person in their care. Most families do better if, once again, they have done some planning before a crisis hits. Shown below is a series of tasks that can be accomplished prior to an emergency situation:

MAKE AN APPOINTMENT

A caregiver can arrange a meeting with a doctor or a member of the clergy before a crisis occurs. Questions regarding procedures, protocols, even legal issues, can be addressed at the meeting. These professionals can be asked in advance about their policy concerning emergency calls after regular work hours.

SELECT A FUNERAL HOME

It is much better to make arrangements about burial plans *before* the emergency occurs. Which funeral home, funeral director, or mortician to select, whether to have a burial or a cremation—even whether to have an autopsy—should be decided in advance. If done properly, only a phone call needs to be made when the death occurs.

DECIDE HOW TO SPEND THE LAST MOMENTS

When death occurs, some people want to have time alone with the deceased. Others want family members close by, perhaps even special friends. It is important to contemplate how you think you would like to spend the last moments (knowing full well that your mind may change), perhaps even making a phone list of people to call.

PLAN THE NOTIFICATION

Many people call 911 when a person has a life-threatening emergency or is near death. Paramedics usually arrive first, and they may attempt resuscitation. If this is not the caregiver's wish, it may be best not to notify these professionals. With such variables in mind, it is important to plan how notification will occur.

BETH'S LAST ENTRY

Daddy's life came to an end January 14, 1993. On Rachel's advice, they made preparations similar to those outlined on the previous page. By June of 1992, Beth's father had been placed in a nursing home. Two weeks later, the nursing home called to say that Beth's father had suffered a stroke, one which left his left side paralyzed. Daddy clung to life for almost six more months, finally succumbing to pneumonia two weeks into the new year. Here is the last entry in Beth's journal, which was written the evening after Daddy's memorial service, held in his neighborhood church.

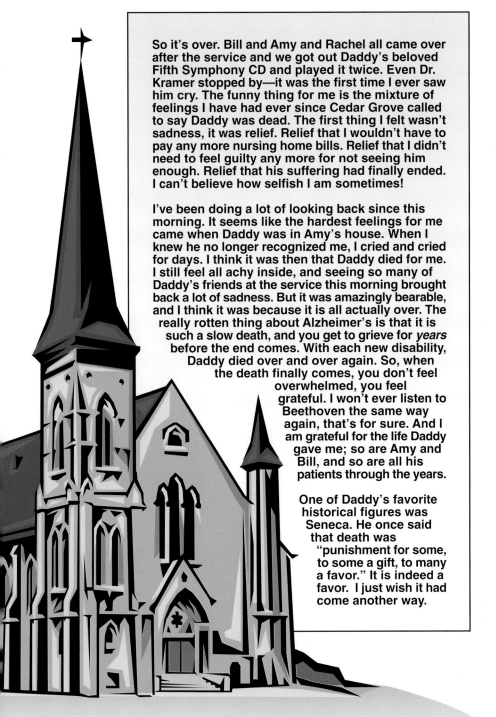

So it's over. Bill and Amy and Rachel all came over after the service and we got out Daddy's beloved Fifth Symphony CD and played it twice. Even Dr. Kramer stopped by—it was the first time I ever saw him cry. The funny thing for me is the mixture of feelings I have had ever since Cedar Grove called to say Daddy was dead. The first thing I felt wasn't sadness, it was relief. Relief that I wouldn't have to pay any more nursing home bills. Relief that I didn't need to feel guilty any more for not seeing him enough. Relief that his suffering had finally ended. I can't believe how selfish I am sometimes!

I've been doing a lot of looking back since this morning. It seems like the hardest feelings for me came when Daddy was in Amy's house. When I knew he no longer recognized me, I cried and cried for days. I think it was then that Daddy died for me. I still feel all achy inside, and seeing so many of Daddy's friends at the service this morning brought back a lot of sadness. But it was amazingly bearable, and I think it was because it is all actually over. The really rotten thing about Alzheimer's is that it is such a slow death, and you get to grieve for *years* before the end comes. With each new disability, Daddy died over and over again. So, when the death finally comes, you don't feel overwhelmed, you feel grateful. I won't ever listen to Beethoven the same way again, that's for sure. And I am grateful for the life Daddy gave me; so are Amy and Bill, and so are all his patients through the years.

One of Daddy's favorite historical figures was Seneca. He once said that death was "punishment for some, to some a gift, to many a favor." It is indeed a favor. I just wish it had come another way.

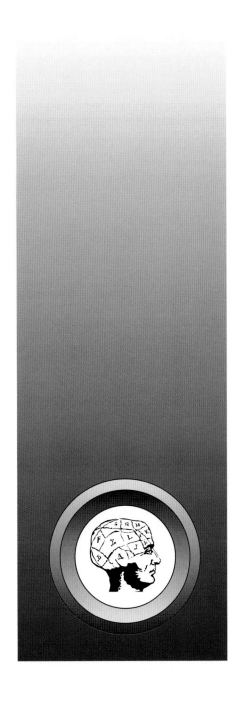

APPENDICES

Other causes of Alzheimer's?

Researchers have hypothesized other origins of AD besides the genetic ones discussed in Chapters 4 and 5. Here are several other ideas scientists are exploring.

As was clear in earlier discussions, Alzheimer's is a disease still in the process of being characterized. We have discussed the genetic data in some detail, but these investigations cover only one part of the overall story. Indeed, other ideas concerning the origins of Alzheimer's disease have been proposed from time to time (for example, viral explanations have been put forward). Listed below are a few other theories researchers are actively investigating. As is true with any notion at the cutting edge of science, most of these hypotheses require further experimental verification, and in some cases, are associated with controversy. It must also be remembered that Alzheimer's is probably a collection of disorders. Thus, even though the symptoms may be similar from one person to the next, the way they got the disease may be quite different indeed.

ALUMINUM

Hypotheses exist that implicate toxic aluminum levels as a source of some kinds of Alzheimer's disease. The ideas came from the observation that aluminum tends to accumulate in the plaques and tangles we discussed earlier. There were also reports that linked aluminum levels in the drinking water supply with human dementia. It was additionally reported that when desferrioxamine (a chemical that isolates aluminum, presumably preventing its toxic effects) was given to AD patients, they showed a decrease in the rate of disease progression.

These data remain controversial. Other studies have shown that high levels of aluminum in drinking water do not lead to Alzheimer's. It has also been shown that AD can exist in people who live in environments where aluminum is absent. Whereas the association of aluminum with Alzheimer's cannot be ruled out, the data remain contradictory.

NERVE GROWTH FACTOR RECEPTOR

Hypotheses exist that link the presence or absence of certain neural receptors to AD. What is a receptor? Neurons, like most cells, can receive information from the outside via antenna-like proteins called receptors. These receptors stick outward from the cell and can bind to various extracellular molecules. One such receptor class is called *nerve growth factor receptor*, and there are two types, termed low- and high-affinity receptors. The molecule that binds these receptors is called, not surprisingly, *nerve growth factor.*

What does the receptor have to do with Alzheimer's? You may recall that the amyloid protein found in Alzheimer's plaques can destroy nerve cells. It has been shown that the low-affinity nerve growth factor receptor can interact with the plaque, and when it does, the neuron carrying the receptor literally commits suicide. However, if that receptor is bound by nerve growth factor, the neurons are resistant to the destructive effects of plaque (see graphic below). Some researchers believe these interactions may explain why some nerve cells are destroyed in Alzheimer's and others are not.

RECEPTORS AND ALZHEIMER'S DISEASE

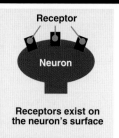

Receptors exist on the neuron's surface

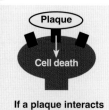

If a plaque interacts with receptor, the neuron dies.

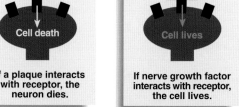

If nerve growth factor interacts with receptor, the cell lives.

Immune system and the environment

Some researchers believe that Alzheimer's may in part be due to the body's natural immune/inflammatory response. In this view, a combination of environmental, hormonal, genetic, perhaps even infectious factors stimulates an ongoing immune reaction. This response eventually results in the accumulation of inflammatory products and subsequent tissue damage. This damage eventually leads to Alzheimer's disease. These ideas form the basis for trying anti-inflammatory drugs to halt the disease.

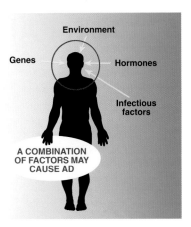

Environment

Genes

Hormones

Infectious factors

A COMBINATION OF FACTORS MAY CAUSE AD

ENERGY PRODUCTION AND ALZHEIMER'S

Some researchers believe that certain kinds of Alzheimer's may be related to energy production inside a cell. To understand what that means, we have to know something about how cells make energy. Consider these two facts:

1) Human cells need chemical energy to do their work. This kind of energy is produced in little capsule-like structures termed mitochondria. Energy from the mitochondria is so vital that if the capsules break down, the cell will die.

Free Radical

Free Radical

Free Radical

Free Radical

2) Like all manufacturing processes, mitochondria produce toxic waste. If the waste is not removed, hazardous molecules called free radicals are created. These free radicals are so dangerous that they will kill the cell if allowed to build up to a certain level.

What do these facts have to do with Alzheimer's? It was found several years ago that energy metabolism is very low in the brains of Alzheimer's patients. Something seemed to be going wrong inside the energy-producing mitochondria. The impairment was so severe that free radicals were found to be building up to hazardous levels, leading to the death of neurons inside the patient's brain. Could this be the reason cells die in Alzheimer's disease?

Later, a mutation in a gene was found that appears to be responsible for crippling the mitochondria, allowing the production of the free radicals. The gene is called *CO* (mercifully short for *cytochrome oxidase*). While it has not yet been proven, many researchers believe that this mutation may be responsible for at least one form of the disease.

Mechanisms such as the ones described here and on previous pages lead some researchers to speculate that Alzheimer's disease may one day be cured. These speculations are considered on the next page.

A cure for Alzheimer's disease?

While there is currently no all-encompassing cure for AD, several recent breakthroughs hint that effective treatments may one day be available to everyone.

"Will there be a cure for AD?" is one of the first and perhaps the most heart-rending question families ask when they discover a loved one has Alzheimer's disease. The question is heart-rending because the answer, currently, is *no*. There is nothing yet available that can stop the deterioration associated with the disease.

It is an incomplete picture, however, to say that the situation is hopeless. Today, more than at any time in history, there is reason to suspect that Alzheimer's will one day be successfully treated. On these pages we discuss several research breakthroughs providing the basis for this optimism. While no one can predict when these breakthroughs will turn into all-encompassing cures, we have been able to slow the progression of the disease in some cases. That alone gives us reason to think we may be able to do so with greater results in the future.

HOPE WITH VITAMIN E

A series of experiments reported in 1997 has shown that everyday Vitamin E can modestly change the course of Alzheimer's disease. The study actually looked at two drugs, Vitamin E and selegiline (a medication commonly prescribed for Parkinson's disease). Vitamin E was able to delay the admission of Alzheimer's patients into nursing homes by almost seven months. The selegiline had a similar effect. Curiously, the effect was diminished if the drugs were taken together.

As you might expect, the result ignited a flurry of new experiments. The ultimate goal is to keep patients away from the nursing home altogether.

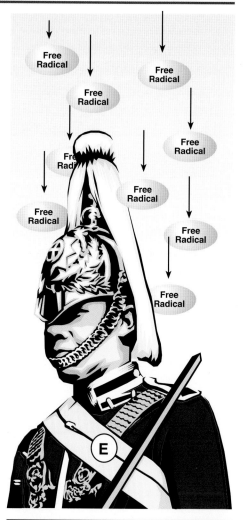

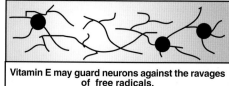

Vitamin E may guard neurons against the ravages of free radicals.

HOW DID IT WORK?

While no one understands exactly why this positive result occurred, the logic for testing Vitamin E has a sound scientific basis. Vitamin E, as you may know, is in a class of molecules called antioxidants. Such molecules have the ability to fight free radicals, those toxic waste products we discussed on the last page. As you also know, some of the symptoms of Alzheimer's disease may be caused by an overabundance of free radicals. If so, then taking some kind of antioxidant might make sense, perhaps slowing the age of onset of Alzheimer's disease.

RESULTS WITH ESTROGEN

Another result that shows promise as an effective treatment for Alzheimer's disease in postmenopausal women is the use of estrogen. This hormone has been shown to have many different effects on brain neurons. Estrogen may even be able to improve higher mental functions such as memory and learning.

With such effects in mind, it might seem natural to ask if estrogen might positively affect women with Alzheimer's disease. Several studies appear to show this may be the case, one of which is described below.

A researcher followed the lives of 1,124 mentally healthy, elderly women. Some were taking estrogen and some were not. The researchers asked the question, "How many of these women developed Alzheimer's?" As shown in the graph below, those women who did not take estrogen had a much greater chance of getting Alzheimer's than those women who took estrogen.

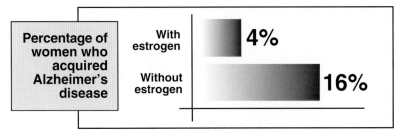

While these results are promising, much more work needs to be done before estrogen becomes a definitive treatment for AD. Moreover, there are health risks associated with taking estrogen (for example, an increased risk for breast cancer). Nonetheless the data with estrogen, as with Vitamin E, represent a milestone in Alzheimer's research. They provide the first glimmer of hope that we may be able to significantly slow, maybe someday even halt, the progression of the disease.

ANTIINFLAMMATORY THERAPY

Some researchers believe Alzheimer's is intimately associated with the immune system. Symptoms may appear because of an ongoing inflammatory response. If that were true, then antiinflammatory medications might slow the effects of AD. This indeed appears to be the case. Ibuprofen (e.g., Advil) is an example of a nonsteroidal antiinflammatory drug (NSAID) that seems to provide protective effect in some cases. There are however some associated health risks with these familiar over-the-counter medications, and even more research will be needed to further prove their efficacy.

GENE THERAPY

With the knowledge that some kinds of Alzheimer's occur because of mistakes in certain genes, people naturally ask "Couldn't the genes be fixed?" Genetic engineering has produced some powerful weapons against other diseases; why not AD? The question is a good one, and in theory, we should be able to treat Alzheimer's with repaired genes. The practical application of the theory to the real world of the clinic is enormously tricky, however. We are probably many years away from using gene therapy as a successful treatment against Alzheimer's disease.

WHAT IS AVAILABLE

What about the present? The Food and Drug Administration has given approval for certain medications in the treatment of Alzheimer's. One medicine is called tacrine (Cognex), another is called donepezil (Aricept). Unlike Vitamin E or estrogen, these medications work by inhibiting a molecule which normally breaks down the neurotransmitter acetylcholine. There can be some improvement of symptoms with tacrine and donepezil, though the underlying deterioration of the brain still goes on.

Difficult behaviors can sometimes be treated medically

Medications can help patients (and their caregivers!) through some of the more difficult symptoms of Alzheimer's disease.

While there are no cures for AD, there are surprisingly successful treatments for some of its more difficult symptoms. Listed on these pages are a few of the troubling symptoms a person with AD might experience, and several medications that may be prescribed to treat them. It must be remembered that every patient will endure a different subset of difficult behaviors, of course, and not everyone will respond completely to every medication. Moreover, different side effects may preclude the use of these medicines in some patients. The names and classes of the medications are provided here only to inform the reader of their existence. As ever, any medication regimen should be under the strict supervision of a physcian.

A NOTE OF CAUTION

Some medications may be harmful, especially if used in combination with other medicines. Certain anticholinergic drugs, or even antipsychotics (see below) could be hazardous to a person with AD and may need to be avoided. An older person may already be under treatment for conditions like hypertension or other vascular ailments. It is thus EXTREMELY important that the patient be under the care of a medical professional, such as a geriatric psychiatrist, before any medications for AD are taken.

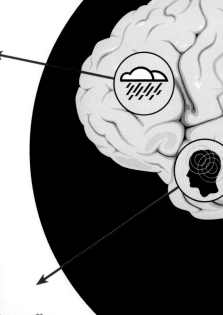

DEPRESSION

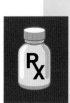

Many Alzheimer's patients suffer depression during the course of their illness. The *antidepressants* used to treat depressed, non-AD patients work on people with Alzheimer's as well. (Some antidepressants, however, can worsen AD symptoms; a person taking antidepressants should always be under the supervision of a physician).

HALLUCINATIONS

Some Alzheimer's patients suffer from hallucinations (such as hearing voices or seeing things that are not there). The class of medicines that can help patients suffering from hallucinations is called *antipsychotic medication*.

PROBLEMS IN COGNITION

Medications exist that may slow the progress of cognitive impairment. Two such drugs are tacrine and donepezil. Vitamin E may also be helpful.

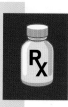

DELUSIONAL THINKING

A class of medications that may help patients who suffer from delusions are the antipsychotic drugs, the same class of medications previously described for patients who hallucinate.

ANXIETY

For anxiety, medications such as buspirone (BuSpar) or one of the *benzodiazepines* may be prescribed. Antidepressants may be used as well.

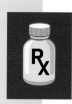

APATHY

Medications exist that may help patients suffering from listlessness or apathy. One such medication is called methylphenidate (Ritalin).

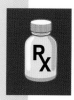

PHYSICAL AGGRESSION

Medications exist that can calm physically aggressive patients with Alzheimer's. Two such drugs are carbamazepine (Tegretol) and valproic acid. Antipsychotic medications are also sometimes prescribed.

Alzheimer's by the numbers

Alzheimer's disease exacts a terrible price, both in human and monetary terms. Here are a few national statistics on the incidence and cost of the disease.

As the Baby Boomer generation gets older, the number of people who will acquire Alzheimer's disease is expected to skyrocket. Related health care costs will rise as well. Listed on this page are a few of the statistics associated with the incidence of Alzheimer's in the United States and the money the disease is expected to cost. If researchers could find a way to delay the onset of symptoms by as little as five years, the health care costs shown on this page could be cut in half.

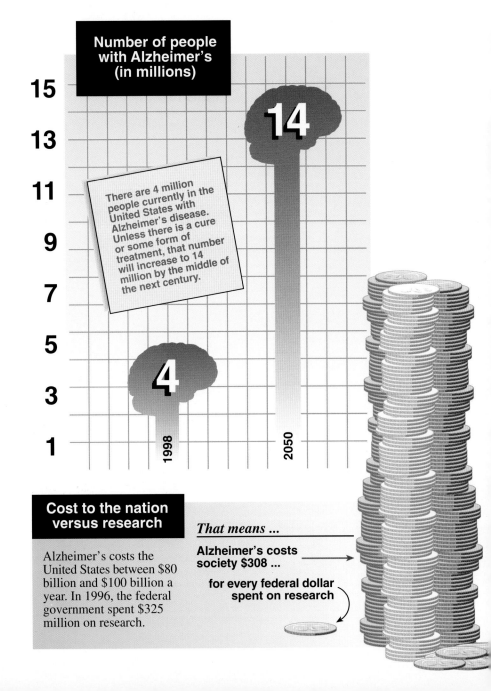

Number of people with Alzheimer's (in millions)

15
13
11
9
7
5
3
1

There are 4 million people currently in the United States with Alzheimer's disease. Unless there is a cure or some form of treatment, that number will increase to 14 million by the middle of the next century.

14

4

1998

2050

Cost to the nation versus research

Alzheimer's costs the United States between $80 billion and $100 billion a year. In 1996, the federal government spent $325 million on research.

That means ...

Alzheimer's costs society $308 ...

for every federal dollar spent on research

COST TO FAMILIES

Alzheimer's disease creates a financial burden not just on a nation, but also on a family. Nineteen million people say they have a relative with AD. More than 7 out of 10 of these patients live at home, with care provided by friends and family. Shown below are the out-of-pocket expenses families pay for the care of a person with AD. Neither Medicare nor private health insurance covers the long-term care most of these patients require.

$174,000

$42,000/yr

$12,500/yr

Average out-of-pocket expenditures if patient lives at home

Average cost of a patient's care in a nursing home

Average lifetime cost of caring for a person with Alzheimer's

RISK OF DISEASE

The costs mentioned above depend on how long the patient lives with the disease. As a person gets older, however, the likelihood of acquiring the disease rises. Shown below are risk data for people over 65 as compared to people over 85.

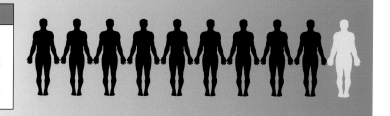

OVER 65

One in ten persons over the age of 65 will acquire Alzheimer's.

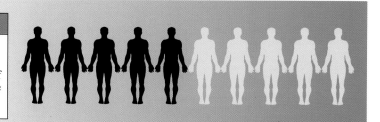

OVER 85

Nearly one in two persons over the age of 85 will acquire Alzheimer's.

What we are learning from nuns

The School Sisters of Notre Dame have collaborated with a group of scientists studying the aging process. Their association has provided valuable insights into Alzheimer's disease.

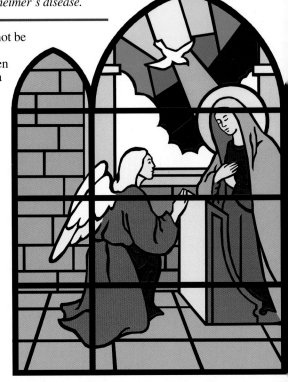

A book about Alzheimer's would not be complete without mentioning an extraordinary collaboration between an American research group and a Catholic religious order. In 1986, scientists from the University of Kentucky formed a relationship with the School Sisters of Notre Dame. The idea was to take as broad a look as possible at the psychological and biological effects of aging. The methodology was to go beyond just the normal blood-sample taking and filling out of questionnaires typical of such investigations. The researchers also asked the sisters to donate their brains after they died. That way the scientists could examine the tissue up close in a group of people they were monitoring well before death ensued.

As controversial as such a task might seem, a total of 678 nuns over the age of 75—and from all over the country—signed up for the research. In the words of some of the sisters, their participation was a natural outgrowth of their mission to care for the poor and for the sick. And so, since 1986, this valuable collaboration has progressed. A nun dies every few weeks or so and her brain is sent to the University of Kentucky. There it is catalogued, photographed, sliced into thin sections to be examined under the microscope. When combined with previously collected biochemical and behavioral information (nuns undergo psychological testing, and even supply autobiographical sketches written when they were teenagers and early adults), powerful data emerge. Some of these data are mentioned on these pages.

OF WRITING STYLES AND ALZHEIMER'S

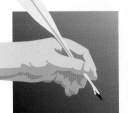

One somewhat controversial study that has come from the nuns' collaboration has to do with writing styles and Alzheimer's disease. The researchers examined the content of writing samples from a variety of sisters, some of whom had Alzheimer's before death and some who did not. They found an interesting, if disturbing correlation between the number of ideas per paragraph in a written sample and the tendency toward Alzheimer's disease. A total of 25 nuns were studied who had supplied writing samples penned when they were schoolgirls. Simply put, the nuns most likely to show the symptoms of Alzheimer's later in life had the lowest density of ideas per paragraph earlier in life. The reason these data are controversial is that they may be predictive. With this information, some researchers wonder if Alzheimer's actually starts early; perhaps the kind of writing content is suggestive of deterioration occurring at a much younger age.

OF STROKES AND ALZHEIMER'S

Of all the data currently coming from this interesting collaboration, the most significant results may come from a mystery we discussed in an earlier chapter. When researchers look at the brain tissue of alert individuals who remained active and intellectually lucid into their 90s, they sometimes make a puzzling observation. The brain tissue of some of these active individuals appears to be as ravaged as if it had been assaulted by a severe form of Alzheimer's. There are the telltale plaques and tangles; there are gaping holes in the tissue showing where millions of neurons have been destroyed. In other words, these individuals are in a classic advanced stage of Alzheimer's disease, yet none of them display the behaviors typical of the brain damage.

These observations were seen again and again in the nun study. In one set of results, there were a total of 61 nuns whose brains had the typical look of someone in the advanced stages of Alzheimer's. Nineteen of these sisters seemed to die free of the memory loss and disorientation that the other 42 suffered.

HOW ARE THESE DATA EXPLAINED?

The researchers studying the tissues of these 61 nuns noticed something very peculiar, an observation that led to a significant finding about Alzheimer's disease. When the brain tissues of the 19 lucid nuns were closely examined, it was noticed that many had a distinct absence of strokes, especially the small ones so common in elderly people (strokes, as you recall, occur when a blood vessel in the brain leaks or becomes blocked and nerve tissue around the area is injured). On the other hand, most of the 41 who displayed Alzheimer's-like behavior before death had obvious stroke damage, the type so missing in their unaffected counterparts (see graph below). This is an extraordinary finding, and provides one of the greatest hopes found to date for successful treatment of Alzheimer's. Medications that can treat strokes may actually slow down the progression of disease—even in people whose brains are undergoing irreversible deteriorating effects (although these findings may be interpreted to mean that the combination of AD and strokes may be necessary to show the behavioral deficits). One of the nuns studied remained intellectually sharp and curious until her death at the age of 101, even though her brain was filled with plaques and tangles and had suffered massive deterioration!

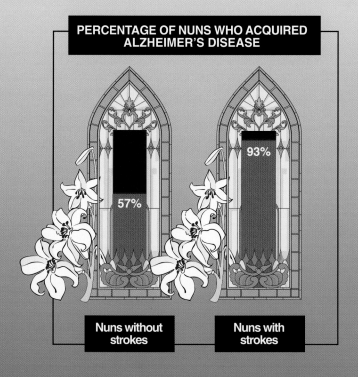

PERCENTAGE OF NUNS WHO ACQUIRED
ALZHEIMER'S DISEASE

93%

57%

Nuns without strokes

Nuns with strokes

Where to turn for help

A variety of resources exist that provide support and information for Alzheimer's patients and caregivers. Here's a summary of what is available.

NATIONAL ORGANIZATIONS

Many societies and organizations have arisen over the years to help families and patients affected by Alzheimer's disease. One in particular, the Alzheimer's Association, has created local chapters in every state of the country (a phone call to their national office can provide phone numbers and addresses of these local organizations). Other special interest groups have arisen as well, as shown on these pages.

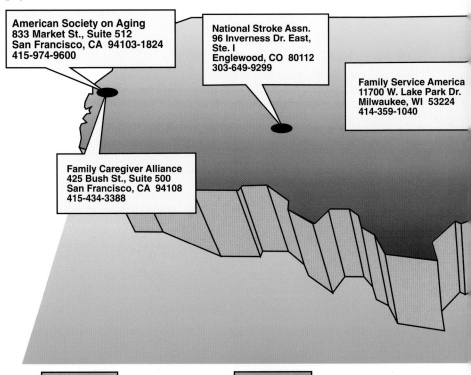

American Society on Aging
833 Market St., Suite 512
San Francisco, CA 94103-1824
415-974-9600

National Stroke Assn.
96 Inverness Dr. East,
Ste. I
Englewood, CO 80112
303-649-9299

Family Service America
11700 W. Lake Park Dr.
Milwaukee, WI 53224
414-359-1040

Family Caregiver Alliance
425 Bush St., Suite 500
San Francisco, CA 94108
415-434-3388

WORLD WIDE WEB SITES

1) Alzheimer's Association World Wide Web Site
   http://www.alz.org

2) Alzheimer's Disease Education & Referral Center
   http://www/alzheimers.org

3) Mental Health InfoSource
   www.mhsource.com

4) Washington University Alzheimer's Disease Research Center
   http://www.biostat.wustl.edu/ALZHEIMER/

BOOKS WRITTEN FROM THE PERSPECTIVE OF THE PATIENT

1) Davis R. *My Journey into Alzheimer's Disease.* Wheaton, Ill.: Tyndale House; 1989

2) Rose, L. *Show Me the Way to Go Home.* San Francisco: Elder Books; 1996

3) Alzheimer Canada. *Just for You: For People Diagnosed with Alzheimer's Disease* from Alzheimer Canada, 1320 Yonge St., Ste. 201. Toronto, Ontario M4T 1X2

Alzheimer's Assn.
919 N. Michigan Ave., Ste. 1000
Chicago, IL 60611-1676*
800-272-3900

*This organization has a network of
local chapters. Callers can obtain
general information on AD, the
number of the chapter nearest them,
or information about Safe Return, a
program designed to help identify,
locate, and help return AD patients
to safety.

American Geriatrics Society
770 Lexington Ave., Suite 300
New York, NY 10021
212-308-1414

Visiting Nurse Assn.
of America
11 Beacon St., Ste. 910
Boston, MA 02108
888-866-8773

National Institute on Aging
Information Office
31 Center Dr., Bldg. 31, Rm. 5C27
Bethesda, MD 20892-2292
301-496-1752

Safe Return
Alzheimer's Association
800-272-3900

National Institute of Mental Health
Office of Scientific Information
Room 7C-02
5600 Fishers Lane
Rockville, MD 20857
301-443-4513

Volunteers of America
110 S. Union St.
Alenandria, VA 22314
703-548-2288

**NEWSLETTERS
AND FACT
SHEETS**

1) *The Caregiver Newsletter*
Alzheimer's Family Support Program,
Box 3600
Duke University Medical Center
Durham, NC 27710
919-660-7510

2) National Institute on Aging Alzheimer's
Disease Education & Referral Center
(ADEAR) 800-438-4380

VIDEO DOCUMENTARY
Complaints of a Dutiful Daughter
(1994) A description of a daughter's coping
with her mother's AD.
Available from: Women Make Movies
New York, New York

**SUPPORT
GROUP
PHONE
NUMBERS**

1) Alzheimer's Association
800-272-3900

2) Alzheimer's Disease
Education & Referral Center
(ADEAR)
800-438-4380

3) Friends and Relatives of
Institutionalized Aged
212-732-4455

4) National Assn. for Home Care
202-547-7424

Selected references

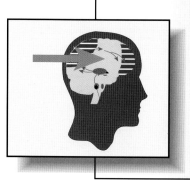

HUMAN MEMORY AND THE BRAIN

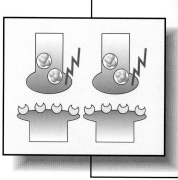

BIOLOGICAL MECHANISMS OF ALZHEIMER'S DISEASE

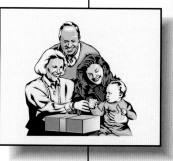

PRACTICAL SUGGESTIONS FOR THE CAREGIVERS OF AD PATIENTS

- Alkon, D.L. 1995. Molecular mechanisms of associative memory and their clinical implications. *Behavioral Brain Research* 66(1-2):151-160.
- Chun, M.R., and R. Mayeux. 1994. Alzheimer's disease. *Current Opinion in Neurology* 7(4):299-304.
- Etcheberrigaray, E., G.E. Gibson, and D.L. Alkon. 1994. Molecular mechanisms of memory and pathophysiology of Alzheimer's disease. *Annals of the New York Academy of Life Sciences* 747:245-255.
- Fletcher, P.C., R.J. Dolan, and C.D. Frith. 1995. The functional anatomy of memory. *Experentia* 51(12):1197-1207.
- Goldman-Rakic, P.S. 1995. Cellular basis of working memory. *Neuron* 14(3):477-485.
- Randolph, C., M.C. Tierney, and T.N. Chase. 1995. Implicit memory in Alzheimer's disease. *Journal of Clinical and Experimental Neuropsychology* 17(3):343-351.
- Rapp, P.R., and W.C. Heindel. 1994. Memory systems in normal and pathological aging. *Current Opinion in Neurology* 7(4):294-298.
- Shreve, S.T. 1994. A primer on memory in aging and Alzheimer's disease. *Connecticut Medicine* 58(6):323-326.

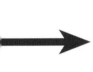

- Edelberg, H.K., and J.Y. Wei. 1996. The biology of Alzheimer's disease. *Mechanisms of Ageing and Development* 91(2):95-114.
- Hardy, J. 1996. New insights into the genetics of Alzheimer's disease. *Annals of Medicine* 28(3):255-258.
- Plassman, B.L., and J.C. Breitner. 1996. Recent advances in the genetics of Alzheimer's disease and vascular dementia with an emphasis on gene-environment interactions. *Journal of the American Geriatrics Society* 44(10):1242-1250.
- Tanzi, R.E., D.M. Kovacs, T.W. Kim, et al. 1996. The gene defects responsible for familial Alzheimer's disease. *Neurobiology of Disease* 3(3):159-168.
- Yankner, B.A. 1996. Mechanisms of neuronal degeneration in Alzheimer's disease. *Cell* 16:921-932.
- Yankner, B.A. 1996. New clues to Alzheimer's disease: unraveling the roles of amyloid and tau. *Nature Medicine* 2(8):850-852.

- Andreasen, N.C. 1984. *The broken brain: the biological revolution in psychiatry.* New York: Harper & Row.
- Dippel, R.L., and J.T. Hutton, eds. 1996. *Caring for the Alzheimer patient.* 2nd ed. Amherst, N.Y.: Prometheus Books.
- Larkin, M. 1995. *When someone you love has Alzheimer's.* New York: Bantam Books.
- Mace, N.L., and P.V. Rabins. 1991. *The 36-hour day.* Baltimore: Johns Hopkins University Press.
- Pollen, D.A. 1996. *Hannah's heirs: the quest for the genetic origins of Alzheimer's disease.* New York: Oxford University Press.
- Powell, L.S., with K. Courtice. 1993. *Alzheimer's disease, a guide for families.* Reading, Mass.: Addison-Wesley.

INDEX

acetylcholine, 151
action potentials, 62
advanced care, 142
age of onset, 94, 95
anxiety, 28
AIDS, 17
aluminum, 148
Alzheimer's Association, 158, 159
Alzheimer's Disease Education & Referral Center, 158
Alzheimer's disease, early-onset, 85
Alzheimer's disease, familial (FAD), 84, 94
Alzheimer's disease, late-onset, 16, 85
Alzheimer's disease, sporadic, 84, 85
Alzheimer, Alois, 11, 12, 85, 96
American Geriatrics Society, 159
American Society on Aging, 158
amino acids, 73, 78, 79, 92, 93
amygdala, 86
amyloid precursor protein (APP), 88, 89, 90, 102
antidepressant therapy, 152
anti-inflammatory therapy, 149, 151
antioxidents, 150
antipsychotic therapy, 152
anxiety, 28
apathy, 31
apolopoprotein E4 (ApoE4), 94
axon, 59, 87
axon terminal, 59, 87
behavior, patient, 110, 111, 112, 113
behaviors, difficult, 112, 114, 116, 117
behaviors, sexual, 124
benzodiazepines, 153
beta amyloid 46, 88 90, 91, 94
biologically based psychiatry, 13
books, patients' perspectives, 158
bruises, 33
buspirone, 114, 153
carbamazepine, 153
catastrophic reaction, 113
cause of death, actual, 36
cause of death, immediate, 36
cell body, 58
cerebellum, 53
cerebral cortex, 53
cerebrum, 53
cholinergic pathway, 107
chromosomes, 60, 69, 94
colchicine, 151
computerized tomography (CT), 19
concealment, 24
constipation, 33
corpus callosum, 52
cost of research, 154
cost to society, 154
cost, average, to families, 155
Creutzfeld-Jakob disease, 17
cytochrome oxidase, 149
cytoplasm, 61, 69, 88
cytoskeleton, 97, 102
cytosol, 61, 69, 77
death-and-dying issues, 144, 145
dehydration, 32, 131
delusions, 29

dendrites, 58, 87
dental problems, 33
deoxyribonucleic acid (DNA), 60, 69, 78, 82
dependency, 30
depression, 17, 28, 125
difficult behaviors, 116, 117
distractability, 27
donepezil, 151, 153
double helix, 60, 61, 69, 73, 78
drug/drug interactions, 152
electroencephalography (EEG) 19
environmental stress, 114
estrogen, 151
exercise, 140, 141
Family Caregiver Alliance, 158
Family Service America, 158
filaments, 101
Food & Drug Administration, 151
fractures, 33
free radicals, 149
frontal lobe, 86
gene therapy, 151
gene, amyloid precursor protein (APP), 94
gene, apoE4, 94
genetic code, 72, 74, 79, 92
heart disease, 37
hippocampus, 54, 86, 107
HIV, 17
hunger, caregiver response to, 129
ibuprofen, 151
immune system, 149, 151
incontinence, fecal, 35, 138
incontinence, urinary, 35, 136
ion channels, 71
irritability, 28
Kraepelin, Emil, 11, 13
legal issues, 143
lesions, 27
life expectancy, 39
listening, 123
Living Will, 143
living quarters, 126
locus ceruleus, 107
lost or hidden objects, 25
magnetic resonance imaging (MRI), 18, 19
mealtime, 128, 130, 131
medulla, 53
memory loss, coping with 124, 125
memory, episodic, 49
memory, explicit, 48
memory, implicit, 49
memory, long-term, 47
memory, semantic, 49
memory, short-term, 47
Mental Health InfoSource, 158
mental status exam, 18
messenger RNA (mRNA), 76, 79, 82, 88
methylphenidate, 153
microtubule-associated proteins (MAPs), 99
microtubules, 97, 98
mitochondria, 149
molecules, 82, 83
motor problems, 34
multi-infarct dementia, 17

mutations, 92, 102
National Institute on Aging, 159
myoclonic jerks, 34
National Stroke Association, 158
nerve cell structure, 58, 59
nerve growth factor, 148
neuritic plaques, 12, 83, 86, 87, 96, 102
neuritic plaques, genes associated with, 94
neurofibrillary tangles, 12, 83, 86, 96, 97, 102
neurons, 22, 82
neurotransmitters, 66
newsletters, 159
Nissl, Franz, 13
nucleotides, 73, 78, 79, 92, 93
nucleus, cell, 60, 69, 79
paranoia, 29
parietal lobe, 86, 107
Parkinson's disease, 17
personal hygiene, 132, 133, 134, 135
phosphates, 100, 101
Pick's disease, 17
plaques. *see* neuritic plaques
pleated sheets, 90
pneumonia, 33
positron emission tomography (PET), 19
postsynaptic neuron, 62
posttranslational modification, 88
prefrontal cortex, 107
Presenilin 1, 94, 95
Presenilin 2, 94, 95
pressure sores, 32
presynaptic neuron, 62
proteins, 70, 88, 89, 92
Purkinje cell, 59, 63
receptors, 66

recreation, 140, 141
repetition, 24
ribosomes, 76, 77, 79
rummaging behavior, 25
Safe Return, 159
safety precautions, 115
School Sisters of Notre Dame, 156
selegiline, 150
side effects, 33
silence, problem of, 123
single-photon emission computed tomography
    (SPECT), 19
stroke, 55, 157
support groups, 159
synapse, 65
synaptic end bulbs, 59
tacrine, 151, 153
tangles. *see* neurofibrillary tangles
tau, 98, 101
temporal lobe, 86, 107
theft, 24
tubulins, 97
University of Kentucky, 156
valproate, 114
valproic acid, 153
vascular dementia, 17
verbal communication, 122
vision problems, 33
Visiting Nurse Association, 158
Vitamin E, 150
Volunteers of America, 159
wandering, 26
warning signs, 14, 15
Washington University Alzheimer's Disease
    Research Center, 158